Beautifully written in a readable style for lay people interested to know more about cardiovascular disease. Does not insult the intelligence of the lay person nor does it talk over their heads in overly-scientific jargon. Quite inclusive and extensive.

Ralph G. Brindis, MD, MPH, FACC, FSCAI
President, American College of Cardiology
Senior Advisor for Cardiovascular Disease,
Northern California Kaiser Permanente
Clinical Professor of Medicine,
University of California, San Francisco

The Wisdom of Heart Health has one clear goal – your good health. Dr. Manshadi wants everyone to feel better, so he's put together a book that everyone can understand. You'll learn to regard your heart – that beats an average of 103,680 times each and every day – with newfound respect. As a cardiologist who regularly sees patients, Manshadi strips away the anxiety of visiting a heart doctor for the first time. From the first page, Manshadi puts his whole heart – and soul – into this book.

Joe Goldeen, health-care reporter,
The (Stockton) Record

Great book for emphasizing cardiovascular health and not the disease! It is for everyone who has an interest in the heart from health care providers to the general public.

Alan C. Yeung, MD Division Chief,
Director Interventional Cardiology Professor

Dr. Manshadi covers a wide range of important topics related to heart health that should be mandatory reading for everyone concerned about cardiovascular disease. Whether you or a family member is at risk, *The Wisdom of Heart Health* provides useful tools to prevent, manage and seek proper treatments. Most of all, the preventive aspects of this book are presented in an easy to understand, yet intelligent way, that nearly everyone will find is applicable to their everyday life situations. We are very proud to have such a dedicated and committed physician on our Medical Center's Medical Staff.

Donald J. Wiley, B.S.N., M.P.H.
President and CEO, St. Joseph's Medical Center

Devoting just a few hours to this book will give the reader valuable tools that are practical, empowering, immediately applicable and enabling. Real hands-on knowledge that is clear and thoughtful, presented in a sensitive and modest manner.

Ernest A. Haeusslein, M.D., FACC
Medical Director
Heart Failure/Transplantation Program
California Pacific Medical Center

Reading Dr. Manshadi's *The Wisdom of Heart Health* is, in all seriousness, just what the doctor ordered. Each of his clearly written and easily understood chapters emphasize the importance of a healthy heart and how we, as members of today's fast paced society, should take control of our lives and protect our hearts. As a former professional athlete I have always been conscious of maintaining a healthy lifestyle and this book provides a compass to help the reader achieve true heart health.

Dr. Manshadi's good work is not limited to the words of wisdom espoused in his book. In a partnership with St. Joseph's Hospital, Dr. Manshadi has generously pledged proceeds from the book to help purchase automated external defibrillators (AEDs) for placement in schools throughout California. We should all take note of his efforts and do whatever we can to carefully treat the most important organ in the body – the Heart.

Kevin Johnson, Mayor of Sacramento

As designer of men's fashion, jewelry, perfume, and automobiles to the most influential and powerful individuals in the world, my goal is to make each individual look magnificent and feel wonderful! Similarly, Dr. Manshadi has created an extraordinary book about vibrant heart health overflowing with priceless information for everyone. A very special human being dedicated to his profession and patients, it is an honor to know Dr. Manshadi.

Dr. Bijan Pakzad, Chairman & Designer,
Bijan Designer for Men, Beverly Hills, California

THE WISDOM OF HEART HEALTH

Attaining a Healthy and Robust Heart in Today's Modern World

Ramin Manshadi, MD, FACC, FSCAI, FAHA, FACP

Disclaimer

The intention and purpose of this book is to offer accurate information in regard to the subject matter contained within. It is created and distributed with the understanding that the publisher is not involved in offering medical or associated professional services, and that without a personal consultation and examination, this book's author does not and cannot give advice or judgment about a specific medical condition or specific patient. If medical counsel is necessary, then one should seek out the services of a competent medical professional. Nothing in this book is intended as a diagnosis for your medical condition, and the FDA has not necessarily approved statements within. While every effort has been made to offer accurate information, the author and publisher cannot be held responsible for any errors or omissions. The ultimate choice to enter into any medical treatment should be made together by your doctor and you.

Table of Contents

Dedication vii

Preface ix

Chapter 1 1
FANTASTIC HUMAN HEART...Where Life Begins

Chapter 2 3
THE CARDIOLOGIST..."Oh I Don't Need One"

Chapter 3 7
HEART DISEASE...Now More Than Ever

Chapter 4 11
SURPRISES...A Sampling of New Heart Health

Chapter 5 17
PATH TO MEDICINE...Destiny

Chapter 6 25
COMMON AILMENTS...What They Really Mean

Chapter 7 27
BLOOD PRESSURE...Low is the Way to Go

Chapter 8 31
CHOLESTEROL...The Good, The Bad and The Ugly

Chapter 9 37
PERIPHERAL ARTERIAL DISEASE...It's Not Just About the Heart

Chapter 10 41
ANGINA...The Sitting Elephant

Chapter 11 43
ARRHYTHMIAS...Electric Heart

Chapter 12 49
PALPITATIONS...My Heart's All A-flutter

Chapter 13 55
CONGESTIVE HEART FAILURE...Not What You Think

Chapter 14 57
LINKS BETWEEN ILLNESSES...Unexpected Connections

Chapter 15 59
GUM DISEASE...Not Just In Your Mouth

Chapter 16 65
DIABETES...Predictor of Heart Disease

Chapter 17 71
ARTHRITIS...Something Fishy is Going On

Chapter 18 73
TRUE MIRACLES...Can Happen *Anywhere*

Chapter 19 79
HELPING YOUR HEART...Patient Heal Thyself

Chapter 20 81
CHALLENGING CHOLESTEROL...Nutrition

Chapter 21 89
DON'T WAIT TO LOSE WEIGHT...Our Outbreak of Obesity

Chapter 22 93
EXERCISE...The Magical Elixir

Chapter 23 97
GOALS FOR BETTER HEALTH ...Getting From Here To There

Chapter 24 101
LET'S DE-STRESS ABOUT STRESS...Seeking a Calmer Life

Chapter 25 107
    SLEEP...Don't Take the Lack of It Lying Down

Chapter 26 111
    SMOKING...Heart Health Risks Go Up in Smoke

Chapter 27 113
    SYMPTOMS OF HEART DISEASE...Paying Attention

Chapter 28 119
    THE CARDIOLOGIST'S OFFICE...Unveiling the Mystery

Chapter 29 127
    TECHNOLOGY ON OUR SIDE...Testing Today for Heart Health

Chapter 30 137
    MORE AGGRESSIVE DIAGNOSTICS...Invasive and Noninvasive
    Testing

Chapter 31 145
    THE DEFIBRILLATOR...Shocking Health

Chapter 32 149
    HUMAN SIDE OF HEART HEALTH...Treating Patients with
    Patience

Chapter 33. 153
    WOMEN AND HEART DISEASE...Equality for All

Chapter 34. 167
    THE ATHLETIC HEART...Sudden Cardiac Death in Athletes

Chapter 35 175
    WINTER RISKS...Tis the Season to be Jolly – *and Careful*

Chapter 36. 177
    ON THE SUBJECT OF SEX...Health Concerns and Erectile
    Dysfunction

Chapter 37 183
MEDICATIONS…The Leading Edge

Chapter 38 187
HYPERTENSION DRUGS…Depressurizing High Blood Pressure

Chapter 39 197
CHOLESTEROL MEDICATIONS…Improving Your Blood

Chapter 40 207
ANTI-ANGINA DRUGS…Taking Strain off Chest Pain

Chapter 41 211
ANTI-ARRHYTHMIC DRUGS…Keeping a Steady Pace

Chapter 42 213
BLOOD THINNERS…The Skinny on Blood Thinning

Chapter 43 217
CHOOSING A GOOD DOCTOR…Good Choices, Good Health

Chapter 44 225
AMERICAN COLLEGE OF CARDIOLOGY…A Medical Society

Chapter 45 229
BELIEF IN SCIENCE…Merging of Worlds

Chapter 46 233
THE FUTURE…Roads Ahead

Index 235

About the Author 245

Dedication

I would like to dedicate this book to my wonderful parents and my extraordinary wife.

I am extremely thankful for my mother's ever constant loving support and determination throughout my life, helping me to become a physician, and importantly, a humanitarian physician. I am equally grateful to my father for always believing in me, from the day I was born to the day when he died.

Lastly, I dedicate this book to my wife for her current support of unconditional love, and for keeping our household and family warm, caring and loving – especially given my highly demanding career and our very active children.

Preface

I've always lived in pursuit of knowledge. Wisdom and insight change our world. They change lives.

The purpose of this book is to offer understanding of something incredibly vital to your own life: your heart. In ways, it literally is the center of your being. Dutifully beating throughout the day without a second thought from you – your heart needs to be cared for.

Many prefer to rely entirely on doctors as sole caretakers of this vital organ. But doctors aren't with you 24 hours a day. In fact, they're hardly ever with you – until there's a big problem. The only one always with you – is you. You are your own best caretaker.

Yet most people know very little about what "makes them tick." Some stick to the old head-in-the-sand idea that "What you don't know won't hurt you." But with heart health – the truth is it's what you don't know that *can* hurt you.

Most heart attacks happen to people who've no clue they even had a problem. This is not the kind of surprise you want! You *want* to know what's going on, so you can lead a longer, healthier, and happier life. You want to know – depending on the condition you're dealing with – that correcting an issue can make you feel *better* than you have, possibly in decades.

I've experienced this time and again with my own patients. It's so rewarding to witness the sheer joy on their faces when they realize they're full of more energy. More strength. More life.

This is what I wish to pass along to you: an appreciation for this most amazing organ. The center of our being. The heart.

After years of conducting my cardiology practice, I made a critical realization: my most knowledgeable patients were the ones taking the best care of their bodies.

By educating *many* people through the writing of this book, I anticipate more will take control of their lives. To this end, I queried many of my own patients as to what would most interest them to learn – what would subsequently help them be better patients?

Almost everyone emphasized the importance of a book that was easy to read and comprehend. That is what I hope to have created here. I've written this in a very accessible way, enabling everyday readers to understand, *better than ever before*, how their heart really functions and how to take the best care of it.

As cardiology can be very complex (hence the compelling need for a book such as this), it is beyond the scope of this book to cover *all* cardiology disease states. Instead, I touch upon the most useful and intriguing issues in cardiovascular care – ones that will help the reader step up several notches in their ability to care for themselves. What I present is easily understood, as well as also highly informative and factual.

Certainly anyone knowledgeable can write on a subject. But it is a book's intent, as well as the background of its author, that truly shapes the result. Given my educational, cultural, spiritual and life experience, along with years of a busy practice, my hope is this will be a book of unique benefit to the reader, their health, and their enjoyment of life!

CHAPTER 1

FANTASTIC HUMAN HEART
Where Life Begins

Folk wisdom places the heart as the seat of wisdom and intuition, creativity and love, gratitude and faith. In Buddhism, the heart is considered to be the center of consciousness. Even the Greek philosopher Aristotle, back in the fourth century B. C., identified the heart as the core of intelligence, sensation and consciousness – further noting the heart is the first organ to form, according to his study of chick embryos.

Aristotle's observations over two thousand years ago hold true today. Life begins with the heart.

Our heart is one of the first organs to form when the human embryo is developing. After just three weeks, the heart is already pumping blood through a network of vessels. It's working to send nutrients to every part of the embryo, so that other organs may develop as well.

It is curious how today, we still attach more meaning to the heart than any other organ. When someone is truly caring, we might say that he or she has a good heart. When we are emotionally moved by something, our hands often involuntarily touch our own chest above our hearts. Consider the many descriptions incorporating the heart as its centerpiece: heartwarming, heartfelt, heartland, hearty, heartthrob, as well as heartbroken, heartless, heartache. Valentine's Day celebrates the heart.

So one might surmise – if our heart is that important to us – perhaps we should treat it just as importantly.

For a cardiologist or a patient – the focus of heart health can all too often be just to cure or prevent disease. Certainly that is a priority, but can there be more? It is certainly more challenging to lead a fulfilling, expansive, loving life when you are having heart problems. It can be done, but it is much more difficult.

A New Approach

Perhaps we can begin to look at a healthy heart as one not simply free from disease and ailments, but as one that works easily and efficiently, dependably and powerfully – so that our entire body experiences greater well-being. This includes more stamina and strength, clarity and alertness, energy and creativity. A truly healthy heart helps you accomplish more in your career, with your family and friends, and in romantic relationships – *every area of your life.*

I find it interesting that many people wanting to be successful in their careers – who spend all kinds of time and money taking courses, attending seminars, and reading books – will spend precious little time attending to accomplishing supreme health.

That seems a bit backwards to me. The payoff of great health – and great *heart health* – is immense. It makes real happiness much more reachable!

CHAPTER 2

THE CARDIOLOGIST
"Oh I Don't Need One"

Not every person sees a cardiologist. In fact, it's not always needed…though once you reach a certain age, it's pretty common and recommended.

Here's also another truth: some people *avoid* seeing a cardiologist, or possibly *any* doctor for that matter.

Yet today's medicine has advanced to a point never before in history. So…why avoid doctors? There may be many excuses, but mostly it's about fear. Perhaps unconsciously, some people feel if they don't see a doctor who might tell them they have a problem – they won't have one.

It doesn't take much clear thinking to realize the fallacy of this logic. If there is a problem – it's there whether or not anyone tells you. And just as logically – if left undiscovered and untreated – a small problem can turn into a bigger one. I encourage all my patients not to indulge in fear when the talk of heart health comes up. It is unnecessary. Too often people only think of the worst that can be. I'd rather they think of the *best*.

The Best?

Absolutely! When our heart and cardiovascular system are truly healthy, we benefit from more energy, alertness, positive attitude, endurance, sleep…. happiness. The truth is, most people have no clue how stunningly terrific their bodies could feel and function, if their health was optimal.

Ultimately, that is the goal. One aspect of cardiology different than most other fields of medicine is that we provide services all the way from prevention to intervention. Compare this to those who are purely "preventative doctors" – those who focus primarily on prevention of serious problems. Or to surgeons, who only intervene once things have become pretty serious.

Cardiologists start from the beginning. We teach patients about prevention, treating their mild issues like high blood pressure or cholesterol. But in more serious cases, such as heart attacks, cardiologists will save their lives with surgery. Then we continue to educate and treat to prevent patients from ever experiencing another such event, and to improve their health to the point that they can truly enjoy life.

It happens all the time that my patients benefit by renewed vigor, capacity and resilience. I recently had a patient come in feeling weak and tired pretty much all the time. He was losing passion for life and becoming resigned to always feeling poorly. The effect this was having on his everyday attitude was obvious. I could see it. His wife could see it.

And his children could see it.

He'd tried all kinds of things to solve the problem. Changes in his diet hadn't made big improvements. He blamed his job. He looked at psychological reasons. All the typical kinds of responses.

I found the cause was his heart. His heart rate was frequently dropping. He wasn't getting the blood flow he needed, and his brain and other organs weren't getting the nutrients they required. I put in a pacemaker (a fantastic device I discuss in Chapter 12), which steadied his heart at a functional rate. He came back smiling broadly, claiming he was a "new man." Soon he could do so many things he hadn't in the past. He was thrilled. I was thrilled. And his wife and children were thrilled.

CHAPTER 3

HEART DISEASE

Now More Than Ever

Despite the core pursuit of most everyone to be healthier and feel better, it must be acknowledged that heart disease is still the leading cause of death for people throughout the world. In the United States, the Centers for Disease Control and Prevention estimates that in a recent year, 785,000 Americans had a new coronary attack. They also estimate that about 470,000 people who've *already* experienced an attack – will have another. Not only that, but heart disease is also a major cause of disability.

It's something we should not and cannot ignore.

Dating Back to Ancient Egypt

So has heart disease always been with us like this? The answer is yes.

And no.

It's true – we're not the first to suffer these heart ailments. Heart disease dates at least as far back as ancient Egypt. Archaeological findings show the ancient Egyptians also believed the heart to be vitally important. Not only was it the core of personality and wisdom, it was believed that "channels" stemmed from the heart, carrying blood and other body fluids throughout the body. In other words, they had the beginnings of understanding the heart. *They also had heart disease.* Recent examinations of mummified bodies, using modern CT scans, show that some ancient Egyptians had hardening of the arteries (which we today also call atherosclerosis).

Jump ahead in time, and we find that Britons in the Middle Ages also experienced heart disease, though fairly infrequently and with few deaths occurring from it. While human bodies back then were no more immune to these conditions than ours are today, the English of those times tended to eat healthier, more natural foods.

The fact is, deaths due to heart problems were fairly rare in pre-industrial society. It wasn't until after the Industrial Revolution (late 18th and early 19th century), that heart disease became more common, and people were more likely to die from it. Before relying on machinery, people worked mostly by performing manual labor. This physical activity not only accelerated blood flow, it also diminished fatty deposits from the body.

What people ate also changed after the Industrial Revolution. Beforehand, they consumed more natural foods, including whole grains and unprocessed dairy. But the creation of new machines allowed the production of less healthy, much richer foods.

In today's world, processed foods have become highly popular. They're easy, often cheaper, and certainly faster (hence the moniker, "fast food"). They've become the first, easiest choice for many. Plus today, people are more sedentary than ever. Machines do more and more of the work, while more and more of us sit while working at computers and desks. Children have developed similar habits of working and playing at computers (and video game consoles). People are gaining weight. Obesity has now become a major health concern.

And heart disease is the number one killer of people. So yes, we *do* need to pay attention.

Cardiology to the Rescue

There is good news along with all of this. Cardiology (the study of heart function, structure and illness) is always transforming and improving. In fact, if you were to look at the medical journals for all the various medical fields – the area where the *most* change is happening?

Cardiology.

In this fast-developing field, there are constant improvements in treatment – for both prevention and for correcting serious problems. There is a growing knowledge base to pass onto patients so they may be *more proactive* in their heart health – to fix what might already be a problem, and for improving health in order to *prevent there ever being a problem*. In the last 10 years, due to all the changes in the guidelines for treating cardiac patients, we've cut down mortality from heart disease *by 28 percent*. That is highly significant.

On the flip side, some factors contributing to heart disease have gone up. Obesity is on the rise. Diabetes is on the rise. That's where there must be education.

That is why I wrote this book. Please be good to yourself and read ahead. Don't be "afraid." *Even if you think you know all about heart health*, remember that cardiology and heart health experience the most informational growth of all medical fields. What you learn will make sense, leave you with much greater understanding and appreciation of your *amazing heart* and body, and provide you with ways to enjoy the best health possible along with the greatest pleasure and happiness.

And yes, it may even save your life.

CHAPTER 4

SURPRISES

A Sampling of New Heart Health

Because more advancements occur in cardiology than in any other field of medicine, good cardiologists are always learning and researching to stay on top of the latest discoveries.

These ongoing, new findings are why you should seek a good cardiologist. Believe me, I'm not saying this to drum up business. I've no shortage of patients, my practice is quite full. But the same reason that impassioned me to go into cardiology – to save lives and improve peoples' health – drives me now to impart this information to you. So you can benefit from the latest science and knowledge in the field, and take care of your heart health.

To illustrate, let me give you some examples of fresh developments in cardiology.

Women and Heart Disease

This is currently a big issue in cardiology. Why? Because it's long been popularly believed that men are more prone to die from heart attacks than women.

So this may come as a shock to you: on average, 410,000 deaths occur annually in men from cardiovascular disease. For women? There are *455,000* deaths annually. (Cardiovascular disease encompasses not only heart disease and heart attacks, but also stroke and heart failure).

It is true, that in general, men develop heart disease 10 years earlier than women. But women experiencing a heart attack often respond more poorly to the event, and those who survive experience a subsequent lower quality of life.

Interestingly, women are much more worried about cancer than heart disease. Yet the statistics support a different view: for women, one out of every 4.6 deaths in the United States is due to cancer. But one per 2.6 female deaths in the U.S. is from heart disease.

So how can this be?

It has been thought that women are largely protected from heart disease by their hormones. Estrogen generally protects the lining of the arteries. It keeps women healthier. *But once women enter menopause* around the age of 50, the production of estrogen decreases. Once that happens, women catch up to men, their risk of heart disease and their risk of dying from heart attacks actually equaling those of men.

Doctors had thought they had offset this change by giving menopausal women hormone replacement therapy of estrogen and progesterone. This was widely believed to help fend off heart disease, osteoporosis and cancer.

But everything changed in 2002. A large-scale, federally funded study found hormonal therapy increased the risk of breast cancer, heart attack, stroke and blood clots. As a result, doctors have become more cautious about prescribing these hormones.

We're now witnessing an increased tendency for women over 50 to develop heart disease just as men do. It simply begins much later in women. I'll say more about this in Chapter 33. Some of the information will be clearer then, as you'll have a better understanding about heart health by the time you read to that chapter. For now – I just want to open your eyes.

Energy Drink Dangers

Something relatively new has become commonplace today.

It's the fastest-growing part of this country's beverage market. They are especially popular among athletes, students, or anyone looking for that extra edge at the gym, on the playing field, or in the classroom. Sold in colorful cans and bottles, available in stores and fitness centers, they are heavily advertised and often endorsed by athletes. Sporting events and concerts are even sponsored by them. The product is marketed as providing desirable and healthful benefits.

And they should have safety warnings on them.

Energy drinks. Beverages like Red Bull, Monster, 5-Hour Energy, Go Girl and Rockstar. People take them to boost their performance and speed recovery times after exertion. Problem is – they can also cause sudden cardiac death if too much is consumed.

The problem? Caffeine.

Almost all of these drinks contain caffeine, which can raise your heart rate and blood pressure. In fact, they can raise your heart rate and blood pressure much more than the actual athletic activity. This can lead to arrhythmias and sudden death. If you already have a propensity for heart disease (which you might not even know about yet), these drinks would further accelerate those conditions. Athletes often exert to the point that their heart rates are near maximum. If they've consumed something that raises those rates further – there is risk. It may be relatively rare, but definitely possible.

Beyond even these acute dangers, energy drinks will dehydrate you – which is not what you want from a drink when you're already dehydrating from exercise.

Most of these drinks are also very high in sugar, though some offer sugar-free and diet versions. Many also contain taurine, ginseng and guarana. Taurine increases heart rate and blood pressure, similar to caffeine. Guarana contains approximately twice as much caffeine as coffee beans.

This is all of such concern that in 2008, the National Federation of State High School Associations strongly recommended that energy drinks *shouldn't* be used for hydration purposes, and not be consumed by athletes that are dehydrated. They suggest only water and suitable sports drinks be used for rehydration. Further, they contend that energy drinks shouldn't be used by athletes who are taking prescription or over-the-counter medicines without approval by a physician.

While drinking one of these drinks now and then is fine, many people consume them far too often. Most athletes would not drink large amounts of coffee before an event. Yet they aren't aware of the caffeine levels in these "energy drinks." My overall suggestion would be simply to avoid these energy drinks, especially as they are not regulated.

In a similarly related subject, let me now introduce the concept of:

Sudden Cardiac Death in Athletes

We look at top athletes as the epitome of the human form. Their bodies have become finely honed mechanisms touting the best we can be.

Until one of them suddenly collapses during a sporting activity and dies.

In the United States, there's unfortunately no clear way to know how often this happens. No one is keeping track. The only way we hear of any trend is through the media reporting instances where some student or professional athlete suddenly and fatally collapses.

There is something common to all of these incidents. All are due to pre-existing heart disease that was never diagnosed in these athletes. It's much more common than people think. Generally, it involves younger people, typically healthy, who don't fall into any of the high-risk categories normally associated with heart disease.

Yet it happens again and again. This has become an area of great importance to me. Not only because I am a cardiologist, but because I was an athlete myself. I will offer much more about this phenomenon later in its own chapter. For now, I want to introduce you to some aspects of heart health of which you might not be aware.

I also must point out that there is much incomplete or misinformation out there regarding heart health. So now it's time to learn the truth. It's time to understand your magnificent, incredibly reliable heart, that beats 103,680 times on average in a single day – without you even thinking about it. Isn't it time you know more about your heart, how it works, and how you can best take care of it?

Let us begin....

CHAPTER 5

PATH TO MEDICINE

Destiny

As we begin, I feel inclined to include this chapter, since when I queried my patients as to what they would like to see in a cardiology book, many requested to know why I became a cardiologist. When people weigh value of advice, part of that consideration is knowing where it comes from. As the catchphrase suggests, "Consider the source."

So: meet the source.

Even when I was a child of five, life-and-death situations were a big issue to me. Profound, in a way. For some reason, I always wanted to investigate why people ended up dying, and more importantly, why we can't live forever.

Suffice it to say, this was viewed as unusual for someone so young.

I'm convinced it began after my grandfather died when I was four. His passing remains one of my earliest memories. I can clearly recall people shaking hands at his memorial service and saying goodbye to my grandfather, after which he was ceremoniously lowered into the ground and people departed. Except for me. I was one of the last remaining. I was eating sunflower seeds and tossing some on his coffin in case he got hungry that night. My parents laughed in a heartfelt way at my innocent gesture. Truthfully, even at that young age, I knew he wouldn't be enjoying those sunflower seeds. But I did it anyway. My way of showing love, I suppose.

Understanding that my beloved grandfather was gone forever touched me, and prompted my thinking about these deeper questions. It was at some point soon after that I knew I wanted to be a doctor. Even then, I recognized the immense potential to help people. That was a huge realization. It gave me focus, purpose and a goal at a young age. I'd become intrigued by the science of healing people.

I'll admit to another factor too – one that preceded this realization – and my birth.

I was considered a "miracle" baby. This occurred in Israel (though both my parents were of Iranian background, my grandfather's grandfather moved from Iran to the Holy Land as a boy). Complications during pregnancy caused my mother to bleed excessively and they thought she would lose me. She prayed constantly during that time. Apparently it worked. I was welcomed to the world.

Years later, she revealed that among her prayers, she had included one for me to become a doctor. She felt that in the same way doctors had helped me to be born, I would assist others in the future. So you could say I was "destined from birth" to be a physician. Even though now a scientist, I truly believe this was the case with me.

While my future was to be medicine, my path toward it was about to change. Because of the war and bombings, my mom took us from Israel to Iran when I was six. Strangely, my life there seemed to foretell my future as well. For the next few years, I was always referred to as "The Doctor." I must have been demonstrating interest even then.

There was something else that set me apart – both in Israel and Iran. I was raised in the Bahá'í Faith. While most are not familiar with its beliefs, I can simply say this is a very open-minded, forward thinking religion, believing in the spiritual harmony of all people. In fact, the teachings prohibit political affiliations or nationalistic agendas. Instead, they support ideas and issues that lead to peace and the welfare of all human beings. As Bahá'u'lláh, the prophet founder of Bahá'í said, "The earth is but one country and mankind its citizens."

The intent is for humanity to live in unity. Toward that end, it promotes equality of the sexes. Independent investigation for truth. Doing the right thing for everyone, while understanding that the quality and ethics of our conduct come back to us in how we will be treated by others. These tenets were all instilled in me at a young age. Somehow it stuck, and would influence who I would become.

Coming to America

Just as various factors seemed to steer me toward medicine, I always felt something guiding my life. This occurred again when I was 12. My family left Iran, primarily to provide additional educational opportunities for their children. We came to live in Elk Grove, California near the state capital of Sacramento.

I was happy to be in America. A dream come true! To my surprise, my schooling years presented an unexpected challenge. I could speak English, so that was not an issue. The problem was that my education in Iran had put me at a ninth grade level. As such, I entered high school at twelve.

But being so far ahead in school, I allowed my study habits to go downhill. I developed a new passion: soccer. My goal was to be a professional soccer player *and* a doctor. *Why not?* I continued that focus through college, where I played soccer and we went to the state championship.

But when I transferred to the University of California at Davis, suddenly the schooling became very advanced. I had to re-tool my lax study habits. This took serious effort, but it paid off. By the time I was in medical school, I'd become a straight-A student, earning the highest scores in anatomy and neuroscience, as well as becoming a teaching assistant. Becoming a doctor was clearly what I was meant to do.

But I was less clear on what *kind* of doctor to be. What would be my specialty?

Again, fate seemed to direct me. As getting into medical school is extremely competitive., you must perform research and volunteer work on top of your studies. At 17, I volunteered at UC Davis Medical Center to perform EKGs throughout the hospital (a diagnostic test to detect heart abnormalities). Curiously, I picked it up very fast. They supervised me as I conducted three EKG exams, and then I was doing it on my own. My very first experience with cardiology

Not long after this, I volunteered to do research for Ezra Amsterdam, a passionate cardiologist who still practices today at 75 years of age. Over and over, he's won the distinguished teaching awards out of UC Davis. His enthusiasm about the entire science of physiology of cardiology truly fascinated me back then.

Though only eighteen – from that point on I knew I was going to be a cardiologist.

Events like these point up how mysteriously life can unfold, especially if you're strong intentioned. I feel very grateful for these experiences that formulated my path. To this day, I'm extremely happy to do what I'm doing. Honestly, I don't know if I would have been as good a doctor in any other field. I truly love

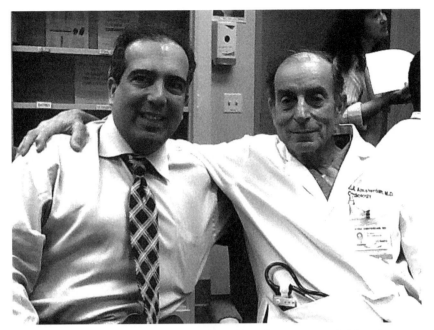

Dr. Amsterdam and myself, still colleagues and friends

cardiology. As many will advise you about careers – first and foremost – choose a field you really like. If you enjoy something, you will learn more about it, you will become an expert, and you will succeed. I was always driven this way. Even in medical school, whenever there were cardiac questions, people would always come to me, even though I was only a student.

But truthfully, my success – or anyone's success – isn't simply due to work ethic. Or commitment to the field. Or expertise. I see other great doctors around me, excellent surgeons who can do anything. They've had fantastic training, with diplomas on their walls to prove it. But their attitude drags them down. It hinders them. In my case, because of my upbringing and life experiences, because of loving humanity through my faith, and because I learned teamwork from playing soccer –

my attitude is one that has helped me advance my life and career.

I truly feel in life that what goes around comes around. As long as your intentions are pure and you help others, you will get the help you need in life. Even with my colleagues and fellow residents that work with me – I always try to help them be better so we're all better. I don't try to take away from anyone to make myself look superior.

A Career in Balance

Today, everyone including cardiologists, speaks of finding balance in life. Often it's addressed in terms of lowering stress and taking time for more enjoyment. I agree with that wholeheartedly. It's something I've realized since I was quite young.

But I would extend that notion of "balance" to even within one's career. In my own field of cardiology, academia doctors (at universities) are highly specialized and able to diagnose and treat rare disease states extremely well. Yet private doctors are possibly more effective in diagnosing and treating the very common disease states, given their greater contact with these types of patients. But if you're only in private practice, it can be harder to keep up with the latest developments in academics. Both types of practices have their advantages and disadvantages.

Today, I'm an Associate Clinical Professor at the University of California at Davis where I teach, while also maintaining a private practice. If I stayed entirely in academia, I would not see so many patients. As a private physician, I'm able to see a myriad of patients and perform a vast array of different procedures.

I'm additionally involved in many aspects of my profession. About eight years ago, I became involved in the leadership of the California Chapter of the American College of Cardiology, after I was invited to serve as a council member. I presently serve as the chair of Media Relations, plus I'm involved in other committees as well. My diverse experiences have enabled me to give high-level presentations about various new technologies and drugs that have come out. Pharmaceutical companies (which play a large role in cardiology, keeping people healthy so they can avoid heart surgeries), have selected me over the years to be their speaker. They instruct me on the absolute latest developments in the field, which I in turn teach to other physicians throughout the United States. This also translates into better patient care in my own practice, because then I know everything that's available to treat my patients.

Just like I encourage my patients, I do my best to balance my personal life as well. Married with three children, I like playing golf (don't all doctors?). Plus swimming and skiing and traveling – when I have time. These days I'm pretty busy. Part of why I like traveling is not just for pleasure, but for learning new things. When in Washington D.C., I relished visiting monuments and learning the history behind them in detail, as well as visiting the National Air and Space Museum at the Smithsonian. I still recall being four years old and seeing Neil Armstrong walk on the moon on TV for the first time.

That amazing image is my first memory of a trait that remains with me – always wanting to know the unknown. It can be learning about most any subject – from fine literature, to notable people like Abraham Lincoln, or even successful businessmen. I find them inspiring, much like I imagine Einstein felt when he wrote:

"The example of great and pure individuals is the only thing that can lead us to noble thoughts and deeds."

Today, I want you to be one of those great individuals. It is my sincerest hope that as I answer some of the mysteries surrounding your magnificent heart and its care, that you too will be motivated to learn more to improve your own health – and enjoy life to the fullest!

CHAPTER 6

COMMON AILMENTS
What They Really Mean

It is likely you already have some knowledge about your heart. You've probably read about various things that can go *wrong*, advice you should take to ensure they don't, and basically, a variety of warnings to avoid getting into heart trouble.

All of that information can be valuable, but most likely it's come in bits and pieces: whatever some news or magazine article covered while trying to grab your attention so it could sell ads, or perhaps an isolated piece of cautionary guidance from your doctor.

Whatever the source, it's likely the information isn't complete. You don't have a full picture. While it is beyond the scope of even this book to cover every aspect of cardiology, I want you to have a more complete understanding of your heart. I'll begin here by addressing some of the common heart issues you probably have heard about, but may not yet fully comprehend:

- Blood pressure
- Cholesterol
- Peripheral arterial disease
- Angina
- Arrhythmias
- Palpitations
- Congestive heart failure

CHAPTER 7

BLOOD PRESSURE

Low is the Way to Go

As adults, most of us have heard a great deal about blood pressure. Most have had theirs tested. Some may even know that when it's too elevated, we call it hypertension.

But most still don't know what it is.

It can be described as the amount of pressure the blood exerts on the walls of the vessels and arteries as it moves through the body. But to be fully clear, when we speak of blood pressure, we're actually speaking of *two* blood pressures. One is systolic and the other diastolic. When someone's blood pressure is described as "one-twenty over eighty" (120/80), the 120 is the systolic number and the 80 is the diastolic number.

Why two numbers? They're actually measuring two different pressures. *Systolic* is the measurement of blood pressure while the heart is beating, while *diastolic* measures pressure while the heart is relaxed between heartbeats.

Most younger people have problems with their diastolic pressure, with their systolic being normal. But as you get older, the arteries become stiff and you have more systolic blood pressure (the first number), while the diastolic (the second number) is more normal.

Studies have shown that if both numbers are too elevated, then both should be treated. That's a change from the standard wisdom of as recent as 15 years ago, when it was thought that diastolic was the only one that needed focus. Now we know that both are very important.

For everyone, an optimum blood pressure would be 120/80. But today's guidelines don't emphasize that as much. My philosophy is as long as a patient can walk and talk, the lower the blood pressure the better (though you don't want the top number to fall below 100). Studies show that even people who just have *high normal* – that is with the top number (systolic) of 121 to 140 – their instance of developing a heart attack is greater over the years. That's why you want to push for a number as low as possible.

Take the Pressure off High Blood Pressure

Sometimes people have high blood pressure and are simply not aware of it. Yet other times, people know theirs is elevated, but since they aren't feeling bad, they don't feel it really needs to be addressed.

They would be wrong.

The truth is, high blood pressure *does* affect you long before you might experience a serious situation. The sheer force of high blood pressure causes dysfunction of the inner lining (endothelium) of the arteries throughout the body. When that occurs, the artery doesn't perform very well. Effects of high blood pressure are felt at the body's "end organs." While most people focus on the heart, other examples of end organs would be the brain and kidneys. High blood pressure can damage any of these organs, possibly seriously.

The obvious question then comes up, "Will lowering my high blood pressure into the normal range reverse the effects it may have already had on these organs?"

The answer is yes – *if* it is caught and corrected early on, such that there isn't much organ damage. Then the organs will recover. The truth is, when you treat high blood pressure, you will always get better. But *the degree to which* you improve all depends on how soon you start with treatment.

Blood Pressure Higher Today than Years Past

It is true - high blood pressure is much more common today. To better comprehend why, it helps to understand the primary reason blood pressure goes up.

Our body has sophisticated mechanisms in place to help us maintain blood pressure in case of emergencies. It's really a survival aid. As a simple example, let's take our cave-dwelling ancestors. If one of them went out hunting and got injured, they might start bleeding. Once you begin bleeding, the volume of blood in your veins goes down, as some is seeping out. But the body needs to keep that blood volume at a certain flow.

So the body has this wonderful mechanism to raise blood pressure. Called RAAS, it's a hormone system that controls water (fluid) balance and blood pressure. Once activated, this RAAS cascade of events raises the blood pressure back up, maintaining blood flow to the primary organs of the body, such as the brain and heart. It is truly an excellent system to counteract against many types of emergencies.

However...

This same automatic mechanism operates when the human being *senses* danger too. Anticipating a possible life-threatening injury, the body engages the RAAS system to regulate in more fluid and increase blood pressure. The stress associated with a perceived impending attack activates this system. The problem is – stress activates the system even when there's no true likelihood of an injury that would cause a blood loss. The body doesn't discern the difference. It just senses the stress.

We hear a great deal about stress today. We're constantly under stress due to our modern lives. Increased traffic on the freeway, longer hours and greater demands at work, issues with family, financial worries, the ever-increasing pace of living...as well as our dietary overindulgences like too much salt and fats and other unhealthy foods – all of this has stressed our systems and led to more hypertension and obesity. (Our modern diets and sodium intake will be addressed in greater detail in Chapter 20).

When the RAAS system is repeatedly over-activated, our blood pressure increases and *stays increased*. Now, if a patient is able to change their lifestyle – reduce stress, lose weight, exercise – they may not need medication. But if the patient is unable or unwilling to make those changes, then they need drugs to counteract the overactivation of the RAAS system.

CHAPTER 8

CHOLESTEROL

The Good, The Bad and The Ugly

Most of you certainly know about cholesterol. Cholesterol is terrible. Awful for the body. We'd be better off without it! Right?

Wrong.

The truth is, cholesterol is one of the building blocks to our cells. Every cell in our body has cholesterol in it, including those in our brain, heart, muscles, intestines, skin and nerves. Cholesterol is also the backbone of male and female hormones, as well as vitamin D and the bile acids that help digest fat.

In other words, we need cholesterol to be healthy. That's why our body makes its own cholesterol in the liver. We need only small amounts of cholesterol in our blood to supply these requirements.

But we also take in cholesterol from outside our body – through food. Many people consume too much cholesterol because of the types and amounts of foods they are eating. When that happens, the extra cholesterol in our bloodstream can deposit in our arteries. This is often a prime focus of the cardiologist.

Genetics Can Play a Role

Before we continue, let me point out that too much cholesterol isn't *always* because of a bad diet. Some people have genetically high cholesterol. Researchers are not sure yet if this is because they produce it more, absorb it more, or from some other cause. Though rare, some people can exercise and watch their diet, but still have *a lot* of bad cholesterol. For these people especially, their only method to control their levels is through some kind of medication, which I'll address in detail in Chapter 39.

On the other hand, though also rare, some people can be obese and not exercise – and their cholesterol is perfect. They're among the very fortunate, and can thank their genetics for that one.

Why is Too Much Cholesterol a Problem?

Though I will go into further detail later in this book, let's simply start here by saying that if you have too much of the *bad type* of cholesterol, it can enter the inner lining of an artery, causing inflammation that may promote plaque formation and lead to blockages.

But truly understanding cholesterol begins with realizing there are three main components to "total cholesterol." They are what I like to call The Good, The Bad and The Ugly.

- The good is HDL cholesterol.
- The bad is LDL cholesterol.
- The ugly are triglycerides.

Because of this, I do not look at *total cholesterol* as a marker (indicator) for having high cholesterol. That is how it was done in "the old days" when someone would say, "My cholesterol is 250." My reasoning is this total cholesterol number is the sum of all your types of cholesterol – including the components of good cholesterol. For example, your total cholesterol could be 250, but your HDL (good cholesterol) could be 80. Your LDL (bad cholesterol) could be 130, and your triglycerides 200.

In general, you want to *increase your levels of HDL*, to above 40 for men and above 50 for women. Similarly, it's best to *decrease your LDL* – generally to below 100.

Fortunately, with new advancements, we can now be even more precise with these measurements.

Going Further – Subclasses of LDL

We now even go beyond dividing cholesterol into its three categories. There are tests today that can examine within the LDL, looking at two subclasses, A or B.

The A subclass is large and buoyant, *and is preferred* as it will not go through inner linings of vessels to cause blockages. But the B is smaller and denser, and can traverse the inner lining of the vessel and cause fat buildup, which can cause inflammation and then blockage, which can eventually lead to a heart attack.

Just to demonstrate how cardiology is evolving, we've also now discovered an offshoot of LDL called LP(a). It's similar to LDL, but can cause more blockages. At this point, the only medication that can lower LP(a) in our system is niacin, which is a B vitamin (which I'll address further in Chapter 39).

Personally, I think everyone should be tested for these types of detailed factors. A person could do a regular LDL lipid panel and have it show that everything is good. But you really want to know which subtype you have within your LDL.

The test is called a VAP test. Turns out, this more detailed blood work isn't really more expensive. It was costly when it first came out, but no longer.

We've now found that even HDL has subtypes, some being most beneficial, while others not helping that much. But at this point in time, these HDL different levels are very hard to adjust, so I don't put too much focus on them. We simply look at the HDL levels. For women, the goal is to be above 50. For men, about 40. If tests were to show less than these numbers, that's when cardiologists advise taking actions to raise the HDL, such as exercising, or stopping smoking if you are a smoker.

So what about "The Ugly?"

Many have heard of triglycerides, yet most still don't know they are basically fat. That by itself can lead to more of the bad subclass of LDL cholesterol. Accordingly, cardiologists want to keep patient triglyceride levels low – below 150. If their levels are above this, patients may be advised to alter their diets, eating less of certain foods, and more of others like fish.

Too Little Cholesterol?

Theoretically, someone *could* have too little cholesterol. We don't know exactly what might be too little. But we can cite that a little baby's LDL cholesterol is only 30, and babies experience the highest body growth rate and are in more need of generating cells than anyone. So you would think that even levels down to 30 would be fine.

Educate Your Doctor?

All these new tests really are a blessing. Consider Jim Fixx, an accomplished runner who wrote the best-seller, "The Complete Book of Running." Everyone assumed he was extraordinarily healthy. Then in 1984, he died of a heart attack.

Why? High cholesterol. Back then, there wasn't the sophistication that we have today to measure the subtleties of cholesterol. Yet even today, some primary physicians do not know the distinctions of the different types of LDL that should be measured. That's one of the main reasons I want readers to learn from this book – so they can take an active role in their own health. Sometimes they have to educate their doctors. Sometimes, they have to change their doctors.

CHAPTER 9

PERIPHERAL ARTERIAL DISEASE

It's Not Just About the Heart

Peripheral arterial disease (PAD) is a condition that occurs when plaque has built up in the arteries that carry blood to your periphery – your head, organs, and limbs. As mentioned earlier, this buildup of plaque is what's called *atherosclerosis*, also known as *hardening of the arteries*. It has that nickname because the plaque can harden over time, and end up narrowing the arteries and limiting blood flow.

It's estimated that between 12 and 20 percent of people in the U.S. over the age of 65 have peripheral arterial disease.

PAD most commonly affects the legs, but can also impact the arteries carrying blood to your head, arms, kidneys, and stomach. Obviously this can be serious – in more ways than you might expect. You must remember that the body is an intricate mechanism. Developing a blockage can have greater effects than even those caused by limiting the blood flow to a particular area or organ.

Let's take for example what can happen if there is a blockage to the kidneys. Many times, I've had patients taking multiple blood pressure pills (each acting on a different body system) who <u>still</u> have high blood pressure. We can't find a cause. But if we use an ultrasound diagnostic on the arteries to the kidneys – we'll find they've developed blockages. That by itself can cause untreatable hypertension, as it actually accelerates the kidneys' release of a particular hormone that can raise blood pressure.

Why does this happen? The answer is pretty fascinating, and very illustrative of the complexity of our body.

If blood flow to the kidneys goes down, the kidneys can get tricked. They think the blood pressure has dropped inside the body, so they release more hormones to increase fluid circulation – by constricting the vessels and thereby raising blood pressure. When this happens, the blood pressure keeps going higher and higher, regardless of the blood pressure medications the patient is given.

Fortunately, even this can be dealt with. I go in surgically and insert a stent in those arteries to the kidneys (a stent is a tiny metal tube placed in part of an artery to keep it open and blood flowing; I address stents in more depth in Chapter 30). That stent allows more blood flow to the kidneys and the hormonal changes reverse. Often at that point, the patient actually has to be taken off all of their blood pressure pills. My advice to anyone on multiple blood pressure medications who is *still* experiencing high blood pressure – ask your doctor to consider checking for blockage in the arteries to the kidneys.

You should also keep in mind that over two-thirds of patients who have blockage in one aspect of their vascular system are going to have blockage in another. For instance, if they have blockage in their legs, they're likely to have blockage in the coronary arteries that go to their heart. If they have blockage at their heart, they'll probably have blockage in their carotid that goes to the brain.

Main Causes

So what are the biggest causes of PAD? That's easy. There are primarily two: smoking and diabetes. Fortunately, you can impact both.

If you smoke – stop. Period. Smoking makes you four times as likely to contract PAD. If you are diabetic, you need to keep a very controlled glucose, with medications. You also need to lose weight, maintain low blood pressure, and keep walking. The worse thing is inactivity. The more you walk the better, even with blockages in the legs. Doing so will actually generate "collateral circulation."

"Collateral circulation?" What does that mean?

This is something truly intriguing. We have blood vessels throughout our legs. There are some "main freeways" that do most of the circulation, plus some "side streets." The side streets are extremely small. That is, until a blockage shows up in the "main freeway" arteries. Then the blood begins finding its way to these tiny vessels, which *get bigger*. The side streets will then carry the blood further beyond the blockage. It's yet another striking way your body assists you.

Varicose Veins

People sometimes ask if these tiny vessels growing larger are what become varicose veins? The answer is no.

Another common question is over whether there's a health concern when varicose veins appear. That answer is no as well.

It helps to understand that veins are "superficial" to the body (meaning they are at the skin level). The blood vessels you see around your arms or legs are veins – not arteries. Veins are very thin-walled vessels that carry waste products to the liver to detoxify, to the kidneys for cleansing, or to the lungs for oxygenation. Then the blood goes to the heart to be pumped back through the arteries, to bring nutrients and oxygen to the tissues. Arteries tend to be deeper in the body and are high flow.

Veins are low flow and fortunately don't get plugged up. But veins do have *valves inside them* that push the blood back up through the body. It's yet another of our body's many unsung functions. However, sometimes those valves become defective and the vein engorges with blood. *That* becomes what is commonly described as a *varicose vein*. Yet there is no health risk associated with this. The only concern is that someone might not like how they look.

Hopefully as you read all this and begin to truly appreciate the truly remarkable body you have, you'll want to treat it better. Honor it with good care.

CHAPTER 10

ANGINA

The Sitting Elephant

When people speak of angina, they are referring to chest pain. Now "chest pains" could mean anything. They can be pains originating from the stomach, from stress, lung problems or radiating pains from gall bladder disease.

But when we refer to "angina," we generally mean pains that come from blockages. Symptoms for men are the "classic" pressure and squeezing on the chest, often described as "an elephant is sitting on your chest." The pain can radiate to the left side of the body as well. Though typically in the chest, angina may also be felt in the shoulders, arms, neck, throat, jaw, or back. If less intense, some describe it as a heaviness or aching, a fullness, or even a burning. Sometimes the person wrongly believes it to be indigestion.

Angina symptoms for woman tend to be different than for men (as are women's symptoms for various aspects of heart disease, as I'll describe further in Chapter 33). A woman might perceive shortness of breath, diffused sweating and fatigue, rather than classic chest pressure.

What's causing the pain is that part of your heart muscle isn't receiving enough oxygen or nutrients (primarily glucose) from the blood that it needs to pump. So to keep pumping, it will use other nutrients as "fuel." Using this less efficient fuel causes a compound called lactic acid to be produced, causing pain if it builds up in the heart muscle.

Not Just Blockages

Angina can happen even without arterial blockages. It's estimated that as many as 30 percent of people with angina instead have a heart valve issue, known as aortic stenosis. This can inhibit the flow of blood from the heart to the arteries. Also, sometimes the blood of people who are seriously anemic doesn't have enough oxygen for the heart's needs, and the person experiences angina.

Another potential cause of chest pain not sourced from a blockage can be due to what's called "aortic dissection." This can result for different reasons, though most likely from severe hypertension that's gone on for a long time, or connective tissue disease. Though not exceedingly common, aortic dissection is where the *inner lining* of a major artery spontaneously tears or splits lengthwise along part of the artery. If this occurs in a major coronary artery like the aorta, and tears down into the heart itself, a person can die immediately. This is how actor John Ritter (of the TV series "Three's Company") passed away.

It's helpful to note that the pain associated with aortic dissection is not the *pressure* normally associated with angina, but rather a sharp tearing pain that radiates to the back. Certainly if a patient feels this, they need to urgently inform their doctor, who can perform a CT scan or transesophageal echo test (described in more detail later in Chapter 11) to diagnose it right away. Then the patient is put on proper medication so the condition doesn't progress further, followed by surgery to patch up the tear.

CHAPTER 11

ARRHYTHMIAS

Electric Heart

Did you know our bodies actually generate electricity? It's not that we can illuminate light bulbs. But tiny electrical impulses are constantly moving through our bodies.

Everything we do – every movement, every thought – is made possible by electrical signals. When we speak of our nervous system sending "signals" to our brains, or our "synapses firing," or the brain telling us to move in a certain way, we are actually referring to these electricity carrying messages between different areas of our body.

The heart is controlled by electrical impulses too. This is the most complex part of dealing with heart conditions. Today, there is even a side branch of cardiology that deals only with "electrophysiological studies." Once you decide to become a cardiologist, you decide if you want to be an intervention cardiologist or an EP (electrophysiologist). I'm an "interventionalist." That means I'm a bit more of a plumber, while the EPs are more like electricians.

Structure of the Heart

Whenever I am educating my patients to better understand the heart, I compare it to a structure like a building. The heart has plumbing, electricity, doors and walls. The plumbing is the arteries. The electricity is the electrical activity in the heart that makes the heart muscle contract. The doors are the valves that direct blood flow inside the chambers of the heart. The walls are the muscles of the heart. Even though they work independently, they are all part of one structure, each part affecting the others. Teamwork. That's how our bodies function, from the most basic cell level up to the whole organ level. It's a subject that has always fascinated me.

The main job of the electrical activity of the heart is to stimulate its muscle into contracting. When the muscle contracts, it pumps blood through the arteries, which reaches everywhere in our bodies. For those who like it a little more technical, the electrical activity of the heart begins in its upper chamber, in a mass of cells called the sinus node. They generate an electrical impulse that is our body's natural pacemaker. It causes our heart to beat without our thinking about it, or even being aware it is happening. That doesn't mean there aren't influences. We can experience certain temporary conditions, such as pain, stress, dehydration or bleeding that will affect this. The nerves and adrenaline (such as from an adrenaline rush) can cause it to beat faster or slower. It is what signals our hearts to speed up when we're in danger.

The signals begin at these cells, then travel from the atrium in the upper chambers of the heart, down to the AV node, a very small area of tissue that conducts the electrical impulse between the upper and lower chambers of the heart.

How do they do that? I like to explain that there are electrical highways within the heart. They go down both sides of the heart – simply called the "right bundle" and "left bundle" – as in a bundle of electrical cells making up the highway. They cause the heart to *squeeze* correctly. Normally, there's this nice rhythmic upper-to-lower movement of the electricity, and subsequent synchronous squeezing (pumping) of the heart. The pacer cells in the upper chamber start the squeezing process, and "give instructions" to the other parts to squeeze in the appropriate sequence.

Who's the Boss? (Atrial Fibrillation)

Arrhythmia is a term that refers to an abnormal heart rhythm or irregular heartbeat. *Atrial fibrillation* (or "A-fib") is a fairly common type of arrhythmia, and is described as a tachycardic (rapid heart) arrhythmia.

As normal pulse rates vary between 60 and 100, anything above 100 is considered tachycardic. Why? When you have atrial fibrillation, a strange thing happens. All the parts of the heart want to be the boss. Every one of them starts firing on its own!

When that happens, it's chaos. The heart starts going really fast. The atrial portion (the upper chambers) of the heart can try to go above 300 beats per minute! In general, a rapid heartbeat lasting a long period of time is called SVT (supraventricular tachycardia – which like many of the long terms that cardiologists use, *actually makes sense*. Supra = above. Ventricular = top of the ventricle. Tachycardia = fast heartbeat).

Now the top chamber can go as fast as it wants and the heart can still function, as long as this aberrant electrical activity doesn't reach the lower part of the heart – the main pump. But if that rapid electrical activity reaches the lower portion, it can cause the heart to pump at 150, 200, or even 300 beats per minute. At a certain point, the pump just gives up. It cannot keep that pace. So you don't get any blood circulation, you pass out, and eventually you can die.

Yet again, our heart is incredible. The AV Node (atrioventricular node) will attempt to slow down these pulses as it goes down the heart muscle to tell it to squeeze. If it slows them down to 100 (or even as high as 180), the heart can still function. It can sustain life. But you'll feel lightheaded, like you're going to pass out.

Two of the most common causes of atrial fibrillation are older age and hypertension (high blood pressure). One other factor is untreated hyperthyroidism. That's why we always test for thyroid disease as a possible cause. If we need to, we'll treat the thyroid disease, and the atrial fibrillation will get better on its own. Sometimes alcohol binges can cause arrhythmias as well, even at college age.

Get Thyself to a Doctor

If you experience atrial fibrillation, you need to be seen by a doctor right away. There are two main ways to treat this problem. One is to lower the heart rate, giving medication that helps the AV node to slow the electrical current going from the top to bottom, to below 100. Those drugs are the first generation calcium channel blockers and the beta blockers (addressed in more detail in Chapter 38). So even if the top of the heart is chaotic, the bottom portion is not going as fast.

Yet even with these medications, the beat is still so erratic that it's not fully regular. It's "irregularly irregular." Instead of the heart chamber squeezing a distinct effective pump, it's more of a weak, non-defined movement. It is as if you were to grab your fingers in your hand and wiggle them. The blood swirls in the chambers rather than being squeezed out. Not only does this produce poor circulation through the body, but when the blood swirls, you're also forming blood clots. And blood clots there, especially in one area of the chamber (called left atrial appendage), can be quite serious. Thusly, the second treatment is giving the patient blood thinners to prevent the clotting.

I recently saw a new patient in his 40s who kept having mini-strokes. He had an irregular heartbeat that was not being treated appropriately. Blood clots would form, get dislodged and go into the top chamber of the heart's left atrium, and then up to the brain or somewhere else in the body. No matter where it goes, that blood clot can ultimately block blood flow to the brain and subsequently damage brain tissue. Symptoms might be weakness in the arm or leg, or the inability to talk. That's why when people have this kind of problem, we put them on blood thinners (anti-coagulants) like coumadin. These drugs dissolve these blood clots and prevent them from causing a stroke.

I had another patient that sporadically had been having atrial fibrillations, and now had a little stroke. We immediately did a TEE test (transesophageal echo), which is the only good way of looking at the atrial appendage. It requires that we put a tiny ultrasound probe down the mouth into the esophagus to look at the heart (sounds worse than it is). I found the blood clot inside this man's appendage. I immediately started the blood thinning to prevent him from having any more strokes.

So patients with atrial fibrillation are treated with medication to lower the heart rate, as well as to prevent blood clots. Then after three to four weeks of treatment with blood thinning (anti-coagulation) medication, we know the clots are dissolved. We then bring them to the hospital, where we make them a little sleepy, and deliver an electrical shock to reset the whole electrical rhythm of the heart. They're back to normal and all is good.

That fixes the electrical problem pretty succinctly. But the muscle takes longer to get better. We continue anti-coagulation medication for another four weeks. Then we can stop it.

CHAPTER 12

PALPITATIONS

My Heart's All A-flutter

You could be anywhere. Perhaps just sitting around, and it starts. You feel your heart skipping a beat.

Now I'm not talking poetry, or about some reaction as your eyes settle on the future love of your life. I'm speaking of physiology.

Sometimes what you're feeling is just one beat. On other occasions, it can happen many times together. Fluttering. Some even describe it as "butterflies in my heart." This is what happens when people experience what is commonly called palpitations.

There are different types of palpations, some minor and some major. Palpitations coming from the top chamber of the heart, if infrequent, are not a big problem. But they also can be coming from the lower chamber. That's more serious, as it would affect the main pump of the heart.

This Premature Atrial Complex (PAC) that comes from the top is a precursor to atrial fibrillation. What happens is that instead of having all the muscle cells acting chaotically, only one or two areas of cells are chaotic. So the body's automatic pacemaker gets confused and resets itself for the next beat. That's basically what someone is feeling. But if it happens too frequently (in the top chamber), it can lead to atrial fibrillation.

You can also have what's called Premature Ventricular Complex (PVC) in the bottom chamber. Occasional PVCs are actually okay. But if they become more frequent, then you start getting tired because your heart is not squeezing well and you're not oxygenating your body.

Can Be Congenital

Occasionally, patients are born with electrical highways in their heart that have "shorts" in them. Or they are born with *additional* electrical highways.

Sometimes electrical signals don't go straight down the highway to their destination. They find a quicker way – a shortcut. If that happens, it disrupts the entire electrical/mechanical cycle of the heart and can cause the SVT (supraventricular tachycardia) that I described earlier. The heart rate can go up to 200, which can cause the person to pass out. Though an issue they were born with, it's not usually diagnosed until later in life, when they're a teenager or young woman or man. It's actually a bit more common with women than men.

When this occurs, I send them to the EP ("electrical") cardiologist.

On the other hand, sometimes a heart has *too many* electrical highways. In those cases, this doctor will enter the artery through the leg, up to the right side of the heart to trace where the problem is sourcing. The doctor will then burn the extra highway with a tiny electrical current. That cures the problem. While the idea of this might startle some readers, it actually works really well.

I saw a young lady who had been to incompetent doctors years before, when she was a teenager. These doctors had incorrectly told her just to take medications and she'd be fine, that she wouldn't need anything done for her condition. Now she's almost 40 years old and has been *fatigued all those years since*. She could tolerate the tiredness somewhat when she was younger, but now she's so exhausted, she can hardly do anything.

I had her wear a 24-hour heart monitor and discovered she had *significant* PVCs – more than 70 percent of the time! I was shocked that no one had ever done anything for her beyond prescribing medication. Since it was an electrical problem, I had her see an EP cardiologist. They went in, burned the area causing the problem, and she's back to normal. She experiences very few PVCs now, and feels better and more energetic than *she has in, literally, decades*. She's off medications and is exercising – and living a very happy life.

The Slow Heart - Bradycardia

Just as the heart can beat too rapidly, there is also a condition where it beats too slowly. Called bradycardia, this state also involves the "electrical highways" in the heart over which electrical activity travels to tell the heart muscle to squeeze. If for any reason (old age, some disease condition) there are blockages along this electrical highway, then the heart cannot send impulses down it. If it can't send these impulses instructing the heart to squeeze, it has a complete heart block and will stop. When that happens, a person can pass out. If not taken care of quickly, they can then die.

Fortunately, this doesn't happen suddenly. This condition builds over time and usually there will be warning symptoms such as chronic tiredness. So when people are feeling continually fatigued, we provide them a Holter monitor to carry with them that measures their heart rhythm over 24 hours. It's like having a 24-hour EKG. From that, we can determine if the heart rate is too slow. Anywhere between 60 and 100 is considered normal. People can still function between 50 and 60, but most will feel symptoms when their heart rate drops below 50. If they're consistently below 50 and not on some medication that might cause the heart to slow, then they're a candidate for a pacemaker.

Setting the Pace with Pacemakers

In the 1960s and 70s, a wonderful device came into use to help people with electrical problems in their heart. Essentially used with arrhythmias, the artificial pacemaker has been a godsend to many heart patients.

Similar to doing a "surgical bypass" for the heart arteries, a pacemaker is doing an electrical bypass in the heart. You bypass the problem of an electrical blockage in the highway of the heart to make the heart squeeze in a normal physiologic manner. These pacemakers are really a type of generator that sends out an electrical signal, causing the heart to beat at a particular rhythm.

Over time, pacemakers have become smaller and smarter.

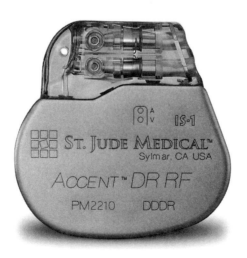

Today, a pacemaker is a disk shape weighing less than two ounces, usually implanted under the skin, beneath the collarbone. We secure one wire from the pacemaker to the heart's atrium and another to the ventricle. The other ends of the wires connect to the pacemaker generator that maintains the rhythm, not allowing the heart rate to drop below 60. Despite how this may sound, it is actually a minor surgery, with most patients returning home that same day. Sometimes they might need to stay overnight in the hospital.

So how long do pacemakers last? That question is really asking how long the pacemaker's battery lasts, and the answer can vary, depending on the patient's condition. Some patients may not need a pacemaker to help all the time, so theirs can last a decade. Others require it to always function, so the battery can deplete much faster. That's why pacemaker patients get routine checks every three to six months to verify the status of the generator and its battery. I've had patients whose pacemakers lasted anywhere from three to ten years.

Though anyone might need a pacemaker, they are most commonly needed by older patients. Many over 85 end up getting pacemakers because their electrical highways are no longer as effective. Some disease issues can also cause these electrical highways to worsen in younger people, who end up needing a pacemaker even at their more youthful age. In addition to protecting the patient's life, pacemakers generally *help the person feel much better*, as their heart rates maintain a certain minimum. As they exercise, their heart rate can still go higher, to meet the greater demands of the activity.

You may have read or heard that a pacemaker user shouldn't stay near a microwave for very long. That is actually true, just as it's generally best not to stand in an airport's security metal detector for any length of time. But if you walk through really fast, it should be okay. It depends somewhat on the type of the pacemaker that you have, so ask your doctor. Lastly, we don't recommend putting your cell phone in your shirt pocket near the pacemaker.

CHAPTER 13

CONGESTIVE HEART FAILURE

Not What You Think

This is a term misunderstood by patients. Despite the name, it doesn't mean the heart has failed and you will die. People can live for many, many years while having congestive heart failure.

What it does mean is that for some reason, whether it be valve problems or prior heart attacks, the heart muscle has weakened. As the muscle of the heart weakens, it doesn't pump as well. You can get backpressure to the lungs and fluids within the lining of the lungs, causing congestion and shortness of breath. It can also cause edema (swelling) in the legs, as well as enlargement of the liver.

The heart is "failing" in that it is not doing its job correctly.

Now That You Know...

Hopefully you now have an improved grasp of many of the core issues possibly confronting those with heart problems. My intent with this, as it is throughout this book, is that this better understanding will wash away some of the fears about the subject of heart health. So often that which we fear most is the unknown.

What I wish to address next are some fairly well-known health concerns that have *nothing* to do with the heart – except that they do.

CHAPTER 14

LINKS BETWEEN ILLNESSES
Unexpected Connections

I always like it when patients have an appreciation of how different areas of our body and their functions are deeply connected. Certainly everyone knows that we use many parts simultaneously to do almost anything. Running, working, even typing at a computer. There are even terms like "hand-eye coordination" that speak to this intrinsic cooperative relationship.

But I'm really addressing how the health of our various parts are interrelated. We know these parts often don't sicken – or heal – in isolation. We've already touched on some of this, such as high blood pressure's potential effect on your heart, kidneys, brain, and other organs.

But some other associations may surprise you. There are certain links between other illnesses and your heart health. Some have a causal connection; others simply a correlation that if you're experiencing one disease, it's a likely indicator you have heart disease too, even if symptoms haven't surfaced.

By addressing some of these associations, you'll also acquire a better understanding of how your body functions overall, and how improving one aspect of health can have huge impact in other areas.

CHAPTER 15

GUM DISEASE

Not Just In Your Mouth

Most people don't think dental health has much effect else-where in the body. After all, we're really just talking about your teeth. In fact, dentistry is its own separate specialty of medicine with its own schools. Dental health is important, but separate.

Not as separate as you might think.

For instance, those thinking dental issues have no correla-tion to heart problems would be quite wrong. How wrong? Hmm, how can I say this clearly? Here: flossing and brushing your teeth could save your life.

Clear enough?

There is potentially a strong relationship between gum dis-ease and coronary disease and even stroke. Studies have shown patients with gum disease have a two-to-three times higher risk of having heart disease. Two-to-three times is sig-nificant.

This is of particular concern, as it is estimated that 15 per-cent of those between 21 and 50 years of age have periodontal (gum) disease. For adults over 50, that number increases to 30 percent. In fact, one study indicated that dental problems such as gum disease, cavities, and missing teeth – were as effective as cholesterol levels in foretelling heart disease.

Three Theories

There are at least three different theories explaining this mouth/heart connection.

One relates to blockage of the arteries (atherosclerosis) being an inflammatory process. One of the normal responses in the body to infection is inflammation. You've probably noticed this when you've had some physical injury and the area around it swells.

Periodontal disease is usually the result of poor oral hygiene, allowing the gums to become infected with bacteria. Those same bacteria can then enter the bloodstream through the gum tissue and travel throughout the body via the arteries. Chronic gum disease can raise your immunity response to a level such that you will have chronic inflammation (swelling) in the arteries. This causes thickening of the arterial walls, impeding blood flow, and increasing the likelihood of arterial plaque buildup. (Though they are the same spelling, plaque in your arteries is different from the plaque that forms on your teeth.)

A heart attack can occur when the plaque that has attached itself to the inner linings of arteries suddenly ruptures (the plaque ruptures, not the artery). Portions of that ruptured plaque stream from its location on the artery and end up somewhere blocking an artery's blood flow. Nutrients, such as oxygen, normally carried in the blood, don't sufficiently get through to areas of the body past this blockage. This can cause a lack of oxygen to those areas, which can result in muscle or tissue death. If the blockage is to the heart, it will cause a heart attack. If the block occurs in the neck (carotid) arteries, that can cause a stroke.

A second explanation for there being significantly more risk of heart disease in patients with gum disease is that the bacteria from the mouth enters the bloodstream because of the gum disease, and actually *attaches to the plaque* in the coronary arteries, accelerating the clot formation.

(You're probably realizing by now that when we speak of heart attacks and strokes, it's really an issue of the arteries – vascular disease).

The third way that chronic gum disease can contribute to heart disease has to do with the heart valves. Again, bacteria from the mouth enter the bloodstream due to gum disease. From there, it can travel to the heart and *cause infection of the heart valves* ("endocarditis"). This can be very serious.

Because of this possibility, people who've recently had heart valve surgery must get antibiotics before having any dental work. Teeth cleaning or other dental procedures can allow bacteria to enter the bloodstream on a "one-time basis." Normally not of great concern. But because the mouth bacteria can go through the bloodstream to the heart's valve tissue, someone with recent valve surgery is more susceptible to an infection that could destroy the valve and require additional surgery. Therefore, antibiotics are a good safety measure.

Plus, speaking of heart valves…

Mitral Valve Prolapse and Dental Work

Mitral valve prolapse means the heart's mitral valve is bulging when it closes. More common in females, there are different degrees of mitral valve prolapse. Some can cause significant arrhythmias from which a person could die. But there are mild ones as well, where a person experiences palpitations and anxiety. If I put those people on a low-dose beta blocker medication, their symptoms get much better and they resume their activities normally. (I speak more of arrhythmias and beta blockers in later chapters).

Interestingly, there have long been concerns about doing dental work on someone with mitral valve prolapse. Anyone with mitral valve prolapse or leaky valve would have been advised to take antibiotics prior to having a teeth cleaning or any dental work performed. The idea was to protect against the possibility of bacteria from the mouth getting into the bloodstream, traveling to the heart and infecting the valve.

But in recent years, those concerns and recommendations regarding this has changed. There is new awareness among doctors and an informed public that the old ways of offering antibiotics too freely can build up resistance to antibiotics in the body, making those drugs less effective – perhaps at some later time when a person is confronted by an infection for which antibiotics are vitally needed. This concern has even extended beyond antibiotics taken *into* the body, to include suggestions to limit the use of antibacterial hand lotions that have become popular.

On top of this, recent studies have shown that few people with mild valve disease, such as mild leaky valve or mild stenosis of the valve, actually develop infection in the valve. Plus, some people may also have side effects to antibiotics that aren't known and won't be immediately obvious. So the advice now is to take antibiotics prior to dental work only if someone has had valve surgery or has significant congenital heart disease.

Strep Throat

Many have never heard of this connection between the heart and dental problems. Correspondingly, they aren't aware how related issues can affect the heart.

This included a patient I recently had in the hospital. Though not an example of someone with gum disease, it was another ailment that one wouldn't expect to affect the heart. A sore throat.

More precisely – *strep throat.*

A very healthy 60 year-old man, he ran half- marathons. He suspected that he had an issue with his valves, but was in denial and never would see a cardiologist. Eventually, he showed up in my office quite short of breath. An echocardiogram showed he not only had a very leaky valve, but also a very dilated aortic root (the first part of the artery that comes out from the heart). He ended up having surgery and getting this part of the artery replaced, along with replacing the aortic valve with a bioprosthetic valve. It was fortunate he came in. Everything went well. He was feeling terrific.

Then about a month later, he'd been having a throat infection that wasn't going away. It was possibly strep throat, but he hadn't treated it with antibiotics and by the time his wife called me, she reported he was very weak and having night sweats. I didn't need to hear more. I immediately put him in the hospital. We found bacterial infections on his valve. By not treating that sore throat, the bacteria traveled and caused an infection in his heart and now he was in some trouble.

After being on antibiotics for six weeks, his valve hadn't improved. I sent him for a second opinion to see if he would need another major surgery – even though he's one of those patients who doesn't want *any* surgery. Fortunately, I was able to sterilize and stabilize his infection. He was doing better, though he still had a really weak heart.

His infections eventually worsened again, but he kept delaying any intervention. I even set him up on a list for a possible transplant, just in case. But it was decided instead to address the valve directly, and he finally agreed. Surgeons went in recently and replaced the *tissue valve* that had been put in (a pig's valve – yes, those are used successfully!) with a mechanical one. The reason: they said the tissue valve looked as if it was 15 years old, even though was only one and a half years since it was put in. This was because of the recurring infection.

The importance of this story is that you should *always* inform your doctor of anything unusual regarding your health. They must know in order to protect you. A normal sore throat may not be a problem, even for a heart patient. A sore throat with a strep infection is another matter. *It needs to be treated.*

This is also true for young children who tend to recover from ailments quickly, due to a very robust immune system. If a child were to get strep throat and you didn't treat it with antibiotics, they could still get better. But later on, it may turn out to have caused mitral stenosis in the valves. This is commonly seen in Third World countries, where people don't get treated for strep. Yet here, checking for strep throat is an easy test that most any doctor's office can perform.

So how can *you* tell if it's worth contacting the doctor to determine what kind of sore throat you might have? A general guideline for adults is that a temperature of 101.5 or higher is significant. A sore throat and high fever (over 101.5), but no runny nose or other symptoms, could well be more than just a cold. It could be strep throat.

Just remember: even if you don't treat strep throat and it seems to go away on its own, you may not be out of trouble. There's a good chance that later it can come back and affect the immune system and cause mitral stenosis. For strep, you want it checked out. You want it treated.

That's me the cardiologist talking.

CHAPTER 16

DIABETES

Predictor of Heart Disease

To the surprise of some, there is a strong connection between diabetes and heart disease. In fact, cardiologists approach the subject of diabetes in a very clear, distinct manner: If you have diabetes, then you have cardiovascular disease.

It's that simple. This is the approach even if no cardiovascular disease has manifested. Why? Because by the point that someone is diagnosed with diabetes, 50 percent of the time that patient has already developed significant cardiovascular blockages.

So what does this mean for the patient?

For one thing, all the guidelines for lowering cholesterol for diabetics are the same as if the patients already have coronary disease. Recent research tells us that all those with coronary disease or who've had heart attacks should aim to have their LDL cholesterol down to 70. In this same manner, if you're a diabetic and have at least one other risk factor – such as high blood pressure, obesity, family history of heart disease, smoking, or you're above age 45 for men or 55 for women – then your LDL should be down to 70 as well.

The interconnectedness between heart disease and diabetes is so strong that I can even determine who will get diabetes, based on the blood work that's normally linked with heart disease. If someone has high triglycerides, low HDL, and their LDL is within normal range – they are very likely to get diabetes, as these are the kind of results that diabetics show in their system. (Though many people think diabetes can be caused by too much intake of sugar, in reality the sugar contributes to the condition, when other processes are in place.)

So a natural question you might ask is, "Do all doctors treating patients for diabetes have them under a cardiologist's care as well?"

The answer is they *should*. But often they don't.

Most primary care doctors usually only refer patients to a cardiologist after some coronary condition has already presented itself. But at the very minimum, primary doctors should make sure all diabetics over the age of 50 have at least a stress test on a treadmill. Why? Because the patient could have coronary disease without any symptoms (called "asymptomatic").

Metabolic Syndrome

There is another tie between diabetes and heart disease. Called metabolic syndrome, this is a set of risk factors that increases the probability of developing diabetes and of developing cardiovascular disease. It's believed to apply to *one out of every five people.*

Before explaining metabolic syndrome, I first want to clarify that there are two different types of diabetes. Their names? Type 1 and Type 2.

I know, not very creative.

Type 1 relates to the immune system. We don't yet clearly know what immune process or virus is involved, but it attacks the pancreas and kills off all the cells that make insulin. If that happens, the patient must take insulin. It usually affects children (it was formerly called "juvenile diabetes"). So if you see a young person with diabetes, that's the type they've contracted.

But if a person develops diabetes when older, they usually have Type 2 (formerly described as "adult-onset diabetes"). With Type 2, the pancreas is producing insulin, but the body's cells are not responding to it correctly. A serious problem, it's estimated that at least 21 million people have Type 2 diabetes in this country.

Metabolic syndrome increases the likelihood of contracting Type 2 diabetes, as well as coronary artery disease and stroke. You are considered to have metabolic syndrome if you have three or more of these five conditions:

- The first relates to size – specifically abdominal obesity. For men, that would be a waist circumference larger than 40 inches. For women, a waist circumference greater than 35 inches.
- The second is having low HDL (good) cholesterol. For men, that would be less 40. For women, less than 50.
- Third is an elevated triglycerides level greater than 150.
- Fourth is high blood pressure. Systolic greater than 130 or diastolic greater than 85.
- Fifth is a fasting blood sugar level equal to or greater than 100.

Usually, you can see abdominal obesity. Being overweight in the abdomen (the belly area) is specifically cited, as abdominal fats in particular can have negative effects by releasing factors that can increase your blood pressure or make your blood more prone to develop clots. Being overweight and inactive and following a diet high in carbohydrates is the main cause in the U.S. A direct consequence of our American lifestyle.

Diabetes itself significantly lowers HDL and increases triglycerides, as well as escalates clotting in the system. Anyone with diabetes should make sure their blood pressure is less than 130/80 (some doctors and/or patients aggressively try to lower these numbers further, but recent studies indicate no added benefit, and it may increase side effects from the additional medications). Plus, patients have to be especially careful to control their blood sugar.

It's really important that diabetics gain control over all these levels. Most diabetic patients also have high blood pressure and cholesterol levels, and together the chances of a heart attack or stroke are at the same elevated levels as patients who've already suffered a heart attack. In fact, a person who has diabetes along with coronary disease is three-to-four times more likely to experience chest pains or heart attacks than someone with only coronary disease.

So – patients really must be resolute about helping themselves.

Medications Lend a Helping Hand

Fortunately, there are several drugs to help offset the coronary issues associated with diabetes.

Studies have shown that even if diabetics haven't yet developed coronary disease, a class of drugs called ACE Inhibition can lower their future risk of heart attacks, stroke, kidney failure and death by *30 percent*. Again, *significant*. If the patient for some reason cannot tolerate ACE Inhibitors, then the next choice would be an ARB class of drug.

Additionally, while awareness in the medical community has increased, some doctors still don't follow the suggested protocol that all diabetics (regardless of LDL cholesterol levels) should be on two other specific drugs. One is a statin (such as Lipitor, Crestor, Pravachol, Lovastatin), which primarily lowers LDL. Studies have even shown that with normal LDL levels, diabetics on statins show less risk of heart attacks or stroke.

The other class of drugs is called Fenofibrates, whose main function is to lower triglycerides and raise HDL. (It also happens that Fenofibrates too, as with many coronary drugs, do a little bit of everything).

I will speak more of all these classes of drugs later in Chapter 39.

CHAPTER 17

ARTHRITIS

Something Fishy is Going On

Approximately 46 million people have been diagnosed with arthritis in the United States. That is a huge number. How does this connect to the heart? Recent research has shown that people with arthritis also have a higher risk of coronary disease and heart attacks.

In fact, studies indicate that 57 percent of adults with heart disease are also affected by arthritis. In the case of patients with rheumatoid arthritis, the frequency of heart disease is much higher.

So why is this? The answer is that arthritis stems from inflammation in the body (most specifically in the joints). In a similar way, inflammation can cause arterial damage and blockages.

Arthritis patients with mild conditions likely have already sought care from their primary physician. Or if their condition is more complicated, they may be getting help from a rheumatologist. *But all patients with arthritis should be more motivated than the average person to be under care of a cardiologist too.*

However, these studies I cite are fairly recent, and not all primary physicians or even rheumatologists know of this connection. Here again, the patient must be proactive and inquire about seeking help from a cardiologist.

A Heart Drug...for Arthritis?

Among many medications available to help with arthritis, a new one may be on the horizon – and it's actually a heart medication.

Lovaza is a highly concentrated source of omega-3 fatty acids, made from fish oils. I discuss this further in Chapters 20 and 39, as it is very beneficial in lowering triglycerides and possibly improving the health of blood vessels.

Yet research also shows omega-3s to have anti-inflammatory benefits at high doses as well. Symptoms in rheumatoid arthritis patients have significantly improved from high doses of Lovaza. But Lovaza hasn't yet been approved for this use by the FDA and the company cannot promote it for that purpose, so I am not aware yet of too many arthritis patients using it to improve their condition. But I have attended meetings where scientists discuss new ways that Lovaza might be helpful, especially considering the beliefs that many illnesses are connected to inflammation. It'll be very exciting to see what additional uses for Lovaza will be discovered.

CHAPTER 18

TRUE MIRACLES

Can Happen Anywhere

As I say repeatedly in this book, your body is an amazing miracle. The more I've learned about it, the greater my appreciation and awe. Everything that it allows us to do, in addition to its ability to ward off illness and even heal itself (sometimes with help), is amazing. Of course, I tend to focus on the heart – the core that helps to nourish all the other organs and parts of the body.

While this admiration has only grown over the years, I want to relate a story that occurred early in my career. A dramatic miracle of its own that took place far from the pristine hospitals and offices of modern medicine.

The First Time

Back when I was a third-year medical student in Chicago, I went on a goodwill mission to a small village in Honduras through an organization called Health for Humanity. The only way to get there was on a small plane landing in an open field or by small boats winding up narrow rivers.

The village only had a very small hospital. Yet early every morning, 50 people would arrive on kayaks from surrounding villages, looking for healing and comfort. There was just one

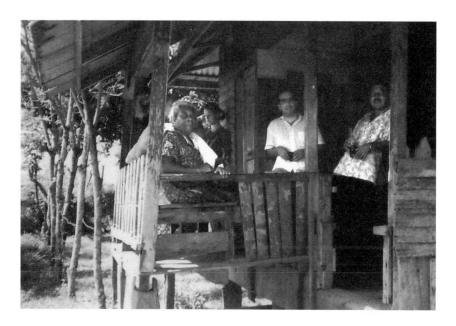

full-time doctor, along with me helping out during my time there.

As you might imagine, treating 50 patients in one day makes for a busy time. Yet between the two of us, we'd finish by mid-afternoon. Exhausted, but loving it. I had incredible experiences there. Right from the beginning.

Let me tell you something about doctors. They learn a tremendous amount in school that they will subsequently need to remember. But one thing doctors always recall without hesitation is the first time they deliver a baby. All medical students go through hospital rotations and will do this. Sometimes it doesn't occur in a hospital and stories can colorful. A delivery in a cab. Or in an elevator.

Or on my first day in this tiny remote community where people lived in huts that could only be reached by a single-prop plane landing on dirt or on a tiny boat twisting up long rivers.

That is where I first brought new life into the world.

Fortunately I spoke Spanish, so no translator was necessary (outside of studying medicine, the best thing I did in my life was learn Spanish in college). A very young couple came in, the woman about to deliver. We put her on the bed and began the delivery process. Though I was supported by the physician behind me, I was the lead doctor. I was totally engaged, nervous and exhilarated. The delivery was successful. I still recall lifting that barely-in-this-world newborn up in the air for the family to witness.

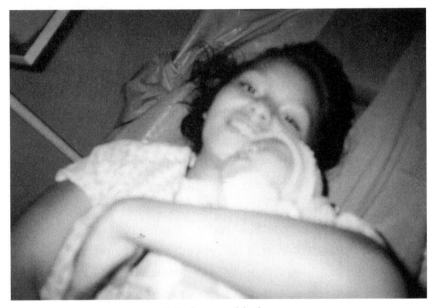

Mother and baby

Later when I began my ob-gyn rotation in a Chicago inner-city hospital, I would have a very dissimilar experience. I delivered 13 babies in one night! It was like a "human production factory." All kinds...tiny preemies... babies that were 12 pounders...babies born with and without complications. Just me and one other doctor – I would deliver, then he would deliver. We'd constantly hear all these many mothers crying and little babies crying. It was intense too.

But seeing this miracle for the first time in the most primitive environment there could be – a remote society so unlike the United States – that will always stay with me.

As will my *second day* in the village.

This was to be a miracle on the far opposite end of the spectrum. My first ER experience in the wilderness. A 10-year-old boy and an older teenager apparently had an argument, resulting in the younger boy tossing a knife into the belly of the teenager. If this had occurred anywhere else in this region, that teenager would've stood no chance. But we were determined to save him, even though circumstances were grim. We weren't equipped to do major surgery at this location. We were too far away to take him anywhere by boat in time, and it was night so planes couldn't takeoff or land. Plus the $300 cost of such a flight to a bigger city was far beyond what his poor family could afford. So that night, the doctor, a nurse and I pooled enough money for the plane. Our goal – help him survive till morning when a plane could arrive to get him out.

He was in very bad shape. I sewed what I could on the outside, gave him antibiotics, as well as intravenous fluids. We took turns keeping pressure on his belly so it didn't worsen. When it wasn't my watch, I'd go off to sleep. But that wasn't so easy. It was incredibly hot and humid, no air conditioning, with mosquitoes everywhere! On the rare occasions I began to nod off, I'd awaken to shrill crying noises. I thought the boy must've died and I was hearing his mother. So I just said prayers for him and finally fell asleep, expecting to be attending a funeral in the morning.

But when I got up sometime after morning light had arrived, I checked in and found *the boy was almost entirely better*! He was in good spirits. He was smiling. He could walk around.

All the crying I heard? Turned out that in this region of the jungle, monkeys would approach close to the village and begin screaming. I thought it was the wailing of people in mourning (guess you'd call that a "misdiagnosis").

This boy had recovered! I truly believed it was another miracle.

Until I returned to the United States and spoke with a surgeon. He said with a knife wound to the belly, sometimes the fat lining on top of the gut can grow over it and heal the wound. He said it could block up that wound even in just one night!

So his healing wasn't the inexplicable kind of miracle I had imagined. But it was another kind – a testament to our astounding human body.

I relate this story so you better appreciate what our bodies are capable of. Even if they have problems, they can also heal and recover in ways we might never expect.

Doctors and medicine can help, but so can you. There are various suggestions and guidance given throughout this book. All of it researched, tested, and documented through science. Heed the suggestions, and make your own miracles. Believe me, it can happen in your own backyard.

Though it likely starts in your kitchen.

CHAPTER 19

HELPING YOUR HEART

Patient Heal Thyself

Though I mention early in this book that some people are hesitant to see a cardiologist, there are others who want to depend *totally* on their doctors. They don't want to change any of their behaviors. They don't desire to improve their health. They just want some pill. Or want to ignore it all…until they have to get appropriate surgery.

Yet, as I have also pointed out, the increase in heart disease is largely due to our own actions – what we choose to eat, our inactivity, and our other modern "health habits." It obviously makes sense that if we had the ability to *cause* much of this, we also have the capacity to *correct* what we've done – if we don't wait until it's too late. Accordingly, new guidelines from the American Heart Association and the American Stroke Association focus on prevention, citing that healthy lifestyles can reduce the chances of a first-time stroke by *80 percent*. That's significant, especially as stroke continues to be the third-leading cause of death in the United States (after cardiovascular disease and cancer).

Each of us has great potential for *positive impact* on our physical well-being – and indeed, our happiness – by making smart changes in our own behaviors. The body will respond extremely well, in ways that can be predicted. We doctors already know what can happen in response to what you do.

Now it's your turn to know.

CHAPTER 20

CHALLENGING CHOLESTEROL

Nutrition

Going over research has brought me to a surprising conclusion: human beings are not really made to be meat eaters.

Animals that consume meat have incisor teeth to assist in tearing it apart in order to eat it. But four-legged animals like deer that are built to eat vegetables, instead have molars in the back to grind their food.

Human beings? We have more pronounced molars than we have incisors or "canine teeth."

Our design being better suited to vegetables, fruits, nuts and cereals – is perhaps reinforced today as people are being pushed to focus more on vegetables and fruits in their diets. We're finding many health benefits to this approach. As far as consuming enough protein, that can be sourced from many beans, nuts, and tofu, as well as various vegetables, such as broccoli.

So do I think this book will create a new generation of vege-tarian-only eaters? I doubt it. But I would encourage people to adjust what they eat and increase the amounts of the healthier foods. Most doctors would recommend this, though I may be a bit more radical in my encouragement. I just feel that eating this way should be the mainstream, rather than the other way around.

Our Diet – Keeping It Simple

Food is a fantastic source of pleasure for us. At the same time, it can also be a terrific source of good health.

While one can go into quite a bit of detail as to what to eat and what not to eat, I like to make it simple for my patients. I tell them to stay away from fried foods. Stay away from red meat. Stay away from high-fat dairy products such as pizza. Why? Because they raise the levels of our body's harmful LDL, and do not help to raise our HDL. Many of these foods also contain large amounts of triglycerides.

I'd also suggest avoiding excessive sweets. Now that might surprise people, at least in relation to heart health. But while it doesn't raise your cholesterol's LDL or HDL, sweets *can* indirectly raise your triglycerides.

There are countless diets mentioned in innumerable books and articles, some in such overwhelming detail that most people can't keep them straight nor adhere to them. That's why I try not to get bogged down in minutiae, and make it as uncomplicated as I can. Now if someone *wishes* for a dietary program specific to them, I'd suggest connecting one-to-one with a nutritionist and creating a customized program. But from my point of view, following these guidelines, coupled with regular exercise, is more than enough.

Yet for those who do wish to take it at least one step further, let me offer some details of a particular diet they can embrace.

Mediterranean Diet

I encourage something called a Mediterranean-type diet. While it doesn't necessarily encompass the entire range of eating habits in the regions surrounding the Mediterranean Sea, we refer to it as a diet that customarily focuses on vegetables, fruits, beans, rice and pasta. This diet has been found to lower the levels of "bad" oxidized LDL cholesterol that builds up deposits in your arteries. It should be noted that most of the grains on this diet are whole grain, and breads are generally eaten without butter or margarines, which contain saturated or trans fats.

The aim of a Mediterranean diet isn't to limit fat consumption overall, but instead to make healthy choices about *which* fats to consume. It highlights monounsaturated fats such as olive oil. Monounsaturated fat can help lower LDL cholesterol levels. At the same time, the diet avoids saturated fats and hydrogenated oils (trans-fatty acids), as they contribute to heart disease. As a result, the diet encourages olive oil as the main source of fat, rather than dairy or animal fats. By the way, the least processed types of this oil are labeled virgin or extra-virgin olive oil, which generally possess higher levels of antioxidant compounds.

This diet also emphasizes polyunsaturated fats, which include canola oil and nuts, particularly walnuts. Tree nuts – such as walnuts, almonds, pecans, and hazel nuts – are naturally low in saturated fat. Do realize that nuts are still high in calories and fat (about 80 percent of their calories are from fat), so they shouldn't be consumed in great amounts. Perhaps a handful per day. It's also best to steer clear of those that are heavily salted or honey-roasted.

The Omega Solution

What I call "The Omega Solution" may sound like the title of a science fiction movie, but it's actually much more real and down to Earth.

Today, great attention is being paid to omega-3 fatty acids. Fish are an important source of these, and a big component of the Mediterranean diet. Omega-3 is good for the heart. At the higher doses, they've been shown to lower triglycerides by up to 30 percent, and possibly also improve the health of blood vessels. For those who don't like fish – or who are concerned about contaminants such as mercury in some fish today – fish oils that have been tested to be free of such pollutants are a good alternative. To a lesser extent, omega-3s can also come from flaxseed oil, soybean and walnuts.

As a result of the positive effects that omega-3s have on heart health, a new prescription drug called Lovaza has been formulated that is highly concentrated fish oil. It is essentially natural fish oil that goes through a five-step purification. I will explain more specifics about its benefits in Chapter 39.

Eggs are another interesting nutrition subject. Today's opinion of them in regards to heart health reflects our ongoing scientific research. There was a time, not so long ago, when the advice was to only eat eggs once a week if you had high cholesterol. But new studies have changed that opinion. Now they say even one egg per day is fine.

Making It Easy

Now with this information, starting a Mediterranean diet is really pretty easy. Buy plenty of vegetables and fresh fruits, while you limit red meat. Eat fish at least once a week, but avoid fried fish or fish laden with butter or heavy sauces. Lemon juice, garlic and other spices can be good substitutes. Focus on using healthy fats, such as olive oil and canola oil when cooking, but still in moderation due to high calories. Eat nuts as a snack. Also, when flavoring meals, herbs and spices can be used in place of salt.

And *read labels*, with the intent to reduce or eliminate saturated fats and trans fats (which may be identified as hydrogenated or partially hydrogenated oils) from your diet.

Red Wine

Much to the delight of many, the Mediterranean diet also traditionally includes red wine. There has been much in the news of recent years touting its benefits.

But it should be noted that use of red wine is suggested only *in moderation*. Studies have shown that low amounts of red wine are good for you in respect to cholesterol. But it's not because of the alcohol. A spectrum of researchers says it's actually the *flavonoids* that are in the juice of the grapes. In other words, you can get the same benefit from drinking simple grape juice.

There are some warnings that go along with recommending wine. If you have high blood pressure or "heart failure" (again, which *doesn't* mean your heart has stopped, but that it's not able to pump blood at an ample rate) – it's probably better not to drink alcohol at all. The harm outweighs the benefits. Alcohol raises blood pressure. It is also cytotoxic (means putting alcohol onto a cell kills it), which is not good for a failing heart. Or if you have liver disease, or have a personal or family history of alcohol abuse, refrain from drinking wine or other alcohol. Also be aware that red wine can trigger migraines in some people.

So, who should drink? I tell my patients that if they are already drinkers, then drink a very small amount of red wine on a regular basis – *only half a glass per night with food*. Any more can increase a risk of health problems, so don't go binge drinking with the belief that you're benefiting yourself. But if you're not a drinker, I would never recommend you start in order to help your heart. Have your red grape juice instead.

Green Tea

Green tea is another beverage on which there has been ongoing research. Numerous articles have promoted green tea and its benefits, with studies showing that drinking five cups of green tea per day can reduce cardiac deaths by 26 percent.

Salt

While we're immersed in the subject of nutrition, I want to address salt. Salt – or sodium – really doesn't affect cholesterol levels. But it *does* affect our blood pressure.

Sodium is needed by our bodies. It's part of our cell structures and is used to affect fluid balances in our bodies. So what's the concern? A diet high in salt causes a response from your kidneys to balance out these elevated levels of sodium by retaining additional water in the blood. This excess fluid stays in your bloodstream and raises blood pressure.

Unfortunately, our diets today are generally way too high in sodium. With fewer and fewer people cooking "from scratch," there's much more reliance on processed foods (frozen and canned), fast foods, and traditional restaurant meals. Today, health recommendations are that people take in less than 2,400 milligrams of sodium per day. For those already with high blood pressure, less than 2,000 milligrams daily is recommended. Yet in the U.S., *average* consumption is 4,000 to 6,000 milligrams each day.

Reasons for this excess are not hard to understand. One Big Mac hamburger contains 1,040 milligrams by itself. Cans of "healthy" chicken noodle soup may easily contain over 1,000 milligrams. Traditional restaurant foods are often far worse. Their goal is to give you something tasty so you'll come back again. It's easy to "enhance" flavor with more sodium.

Depending on the food and the sauce that may drench it – a single meal or even side dish can exceed 3,000 to 4,000 mg of sodium!

So be conscious of your salt intake. If you already have high blood pressure, especially limit fast food or restaurant meals, or choose ones lower in salt (some restaurant menus designate these). When eating at home, don't reach for the saltshaker out of habit. Sometimes we use so much salt, we hardly taste the food. Reacquaint yourself with the subtle and exquisite flavors of your food – and with what healthy eating can authentically feel like!

Never Too Early

While young people may seem to eat most anything with few ill effects (at least compared to those who are older), new research reaffirms that having healthy heart habits when one is young can have health benefits later in life.

It has been clearly determined that heart disease can begin developing during childhood. New research now even specifies that conditions such as abnormal cholesterol levels or hypertension in children might be connected to a higher likelihood of carotid intima media thickness when they are even just young adults (carotid intima media thickness is considered a precursor to heart attacks and strokes). Along with this, is a connection established between low consumption of vegetables and fruits in childhood and a higher risk of atherosclerosis later on.

So begin healthy habits early on for your children. They will physically benefit, and you'll be establishing a healthy lifestyle for them. Having that already in place is certainly easier than their having to transform life-long bad health habits into good ones later on – in order to correct some condition.

Today we put so much emphasis on our children getting a good education and start in life. So do them another big favor – and start them on a life of good health, energy, and happiness.

CHAPTER 21

DON'T WAIT TO LOSE WEIGHT

Our Outbreak of Obesity

Today there is a new "epidemic" confronting people's health. It's yet another of our own creation.

Obesity.

Much attention has been given to the rampant frequency of people now being overweight, starting at younger and younger ages. In fact, rates of obesity have *more than tripled* amongst children over the past 30 years. Today, almost one in five children between the ages of two and nineteen is obese, with almost a third considered to be overweight.

For many of us, this is due to our sedentary nature: sitting behind desks, sitting behind the wheel of a car, sitting watching television or playing video games, sitting while eating too much food. We don't get the physical exercise we should, nor eat the foods we must. Busy as we are today, that drive-thru meal is awfully convenient.

But being overweight is an obvious indicator of poor health habits in relationship to heart disease, with a greater chance for atherosclerosis. In fact, a recent study showed that simply being overweight (not even obese) can more frequently lead to deaths from cardiovascular disease. Similarly, researchers have determined that a child's waist size may reveal more about their cardiovascular health than what's even found by measuring height, weight and body mass index – which is beyond what most parents can or will do. Since more children today are becoming overweight or obese, this simple method might prove useful in helping to identify which children may have an elevated risk of heart disease, such that parents and pediatricians can intercede early and avert the disease.

Again, it comes down to diet and exercise. In fact, studies have shown that for people with illnesses like heart disease, cardiovascular disease, and emphysema – the *single most important predictor of survival is their activity level.* So even if you have difficulties with exercise, under the supervision of your doctor, you should be active at whatever level you can. Anything is truly better than nothing.

Now I should point out that there is something called "morbid obesity." This essentially means bad genes. People with this can't help but be overweight. Dieting and exercise won't fix it . So doctors are doing gastric bypass surgery. I admit being initially against this, but now am all for it. This gastric bypass reduces the size of the stomach so the person gets full quicker, thereby eating less. In this way, someone weighing 400 pounds can lose 200 of those pounds. Plus, along with the weight, they totally lose their diabetes, their hypertension, and other ailments.

Because it is otherwise so hard for the morbidly obese to diet and exercise (if they can even exercise while being that overweight), many today are choosing this surgical procedure. While no surgery is 100 percent safe, I think it is advisable for them. You must always weigh the risks and benefits of anything you do in life. This can include even taking certain medications (most have some side effects), exercise (which can even pose some risk), or anything else you do. But if those people don't take the chance with that surgery, there's significant concern they may not otherwise live long.

Yet if one is simply obese, but not morbid obese, following a diet, *with exercise,* is a much better way to lose weight.

CHAPTER 22

EXERCISE!

The Magical Elixir

In generations past, the population had greater amounts of physical activity.

A high percentage of working adults did manual labor, be it in the fields or elsewhere, as opposed to today where so many are deskbound. Children would go out and play, rain or shine, warm or cold. They didn't rely on computers or TVs or video games for their entertainment. Progress has been great for society. But in some ways – not for heart health.

The bottom line for good heart health is exercise. *I believe it is truly the key,* even more than diet. Please realize that I'm speaking of moderate exercise (I don't believe in extremes in anything in life). It's so simple. When you have moderate exercise, the heart becomes much healthier. When the heart is healthier, its owner enjoys an improved and happier life.

Sure, you say. That makes sense. You already kind of know this.

But do you know why?

One basic reason is that when you exercise and your body is in shape, your heart doesn't have to work as hard. With one pump of the heart muscle, you're able to send enough oxygen and nutrients to the rest of the body, rather than five pumps for someone who hasn't exercised. The heart is working more efficiently. Plus, those who don't exercise use up more nutrients in their day-to-day living. So the heart again has to work harder to achieve the same goals in maintaining the body.

This is why people who exercise have much lower heart rates than those who don't.

Hormonal Release

The other positive aspect of exercise is hormonal release from the exertion. This causes the inner lining of the blood vessels – the endothelium – to become much healthier. I tell my patients that the first thing that goes bad, before you ever develop any blockage, is the vessel's inner linings becoming dysfunctional. How? Mainly through the body's nitric oxide not functioning as it should. Nitric oxide is naturally produced in the body, and helps maintain elasticity of the vessel and assists the artery to dilate (open up). The better the elasticity of the vessel, the better it performs.

This is a big factor in those that develop heart disease. As the function of the nitric oxide goes down, it's much easier to develop atherosclerosis. Why? If the inner linings of your arteries are not healthy, the cholesterol can stick on the walls and cause inflammation.

If you can, imagine a clean roadway where cars move through smoothly, versus a roadway strewn with garbage on it that slows or blocks them. That in a way is what happens with cholesterol. Subsequently, when LDL (bad cholesterol) travels through the arteries, if the inner lining isn't smooth and has debris, the LDL adheres much easier and you get plaque buildup in the artery. Not only that, when the vessel's inner linings don't function well, it leaves them more vulnerable to damage, making it easier for the LDL particles to go *beneath* the endothelium to cause inflammation and start developing blockages. That is what creates atherosclerosis. Eventually, you'll be in bad shape and vulnerable to a heart attack and subsequent organ damage.

Fortunately, if you exercise moderately, the inner linings of the vessels function much more smoothly. The more you exercise, the more you release nitric oxide.

The bottom line is that those who exercise more have lower blood pressure as the inner linings function better. Plus, their weight goes down.

True Tale of Taking Charge

I had a young male patient in his 30s who had high blood pressure and didn't want to take drugs.

I told him, "Your condition right now requires that I have you on medication. But if you lose weight and you exercise, you may not need to continue the blood pressure pills. However, you first have to prove to me that you can maintain that kind of program. Once you do, then I can slowly take you off the medication."

He liked the idea and committed to it. I saw him a month later and the change was already remarkable. He was running five miles a day, five days a week. He had dropped his weight by 20 pounds. I halved his medication. He came in a month after that, by which time he'd lost another 10 pounds, was exercising and maintaining normal blood pressure. Stopping his medication, I saw him again in another month. Now totally off medication – his blood pressure remains normal.

I want to point out that five miles a day, five times a week is really moderate approaching high levels of exercise. Most cardiologists recommend something less intense – closer to 30 minutes, three times a week. Personally, I prefer to recommend at least 30 minutes – five days a week.

Choosing to Exercise

So what type of exercise is recommended? If your body can handle it, running will give more benefit than walking. But walking is still beneficial. Again, any exercise is better than none. The goal is to raise your heart rate during exercise at least to 80 to 85 percent of your predicted *maximum heart rate* and maintain it for about half an hour.

You might ask, "How do I know my maximum?"

Fortunately, there's an easy formula. Simply take the number 220 and subtract your age. That means 220 minus how old you are. Then take 80 to 85 percent of that number as your target heart rate to maintain while exercising. Keeping your heart rate at that level, five days a week, will give you the most benefit. Running will certainly do this. If walking, a faster pace and/or going uphill will increase that heart rate as well. You simply need to find the right exercise for you and *your* body. Of course, you should discuss this with your doctor.

Unfortunately, many people do not want to work hard to lose weight, nor do they want to exercise. Or they don't have the time. Or they might have orthopedic issues and just can't exercise.

Those people will be taking medication.

CHAPTER 23

GOALS FOR BETTER HEALTH

Getting From Here To There

I returned not so long ago to one of my alma maters to give the keynote speech to a college graduating class. There were many things I could have told them. But I chose to explain that I firmly believe the key to success in life is to always put a goal in front of you.

Before you make a decision what that goal will be, really think about it. But once you've made that choice, don't look back. Get it done. Keep that final goal in front of you and remain focused. The road may get you there in unexpected ways. It may not always be easy. But don't let anything keep you from it

Those who are unsuccessful are the people that give up. Sometimes they confront a challenging obstacle and decide this means their goal can't be accomplished. They can be extremely smart people, but they either don't have the drive or the persistence. They quit. But obstacles are part of life. Difficulties and delays will undoubtedly be encountered.

If it was all so very easy – you wouldn't need to make it a goal.

In my own experience, I would never give up. Even becoming a doctor was a tough path for me. I was very young when I entered college at only 16. As said earlier, my life goal then was to be a physician and a professional soccer player. In fact, I successfully played soccer in college, but my grades suffered as a result. I realized I wouldn't achieve my main goal to be a doctor. So I gave up the soccer, and then had an uphill battle to markedly improve my grades, to make up for the average ones I'd already earned while dividing my time up with soccer. Later in medical school in Chicago, other challenges surfaced, including one when I was snowed in and arrived late to an exam. I didn't do very well. But I was determined. I really needed to prove myself. So I focused, and by the time of my last exam at the end of the course, I ended up with the highest score in class.

While these were only some of the hurdles to becoming the doctor who is now writing this book, my patients can have far greater ones.

One woman came in with a major heart attack. I opened up her blocked artery to prevent her from dying. But her heart was severely damaged. After a few months, she was back in the hospital with extremely low blood pressure. Her heart was failing, and it was an enduring battle employing numerous drugs to keep up her blood pressure. But I wasn't willing to give up. Because of that perseverance, and my devotion to knowing everything going on in my field, I knew there was only one chance for her (she couldn't get a transplant because she had high antibody titers).

I sent her to the California Pacific Medical Center in San Francisco. I had done my internship there, and knew that Dr. Ernest Haeusslein could offer her the latest and the best. I remembered that members of royal families from around the globe would come there to receive their medical care.

There my patient received a HeartMate II. At the time, it was only available through research. Called a LVAD (Left

Ventricular Assist Device), this device was implanted in her – similar to how a pacemaker would be. It took over the heart function, pushing blood through her heart via its own pump mechanism.

She was the first person in Northern California to receive one. Because of this, she's been interviewed many times, and many times has voiced that she is only alive because I would never give up. The truth is, she never gave up either. She went through a lot and could have protested, "Doctor, it's too much. I have to quit." But she didn't and it has paid off. She is still alive today, four years later.

So I want to say this: if this woman could commit to doing all that she did to restore and keep her health, to be here for her loved ones, for her life – certainly you can at least commit to eating a healthier diet. Certainly you can commit to exercising.

Not only will it make your heart and body healthier – it will feel great! You'll have more energy, more stamina, more focus, and more pleasure.

You benefit in every way!

CHAPTER 24

LET'S DE-STRESS ABOUT STRESS

Seeking a Calmer Life

In recent years, much media attention has been focused on stress. This is with good reason.

Stress can affect our health and enjoyment of life in profound ways. I cannot overemphasize this point. While many wish to reduce stress in their lives, people today are busier, move at a faster pace, and try to accomplish more professionally and personally than ever before. It's become such a part of our culture that for some, unless they're *overbooked* – they feel they're underachieving.

Some of this increased pace is due to our new technological advances. The advent of smartphones, computers, Internet and email were supposed to make our lives easier and provide us with more leisure time. It's been the opposite. Rather than relax during the day or while driving in the car, people are making calls, answering calls and returning calls. They're texting and emailing (risky while driving!). At work, we're expected to accomplish more and more in less and less time, as we try to keep pace with the lightning speeds of all our electronic "helpers."

There are other stressors aside from the velocity of life. We still have the traditional ones, such as career, relationships, parenting, financial worries, and health. The list is as long as the different lives that people lead.

Two Types of People

There are two main types of people in relationship to stress. By that, I mean there are those that let it out – and those that hold it in.

The main ways we let it out? Shouting or exercise. The healthier of these two would be exercise…rather than screaming and upsetting others around you.

But if you don't let it out, holding onto stress will manifest itself somehow within the body. Our brains will even play tricks on our bodies, as stress can affect our cognitive function. If the brain is stressed, it can perceive pain someplace in the body where nothing is actually occurring. Psychosomatic. But that doesn't mean you're imagining it. Every part of our body has nerves that eventually go up to the brain. The pain is real! It can shoot off anywhere. There might be nothing at all wrong with the hand, but the brain perceives pain coming from there. Same with the foot, elbow…almost anywhere.

A classic situation is someone having chest pains when there are no risk factors present. The pain can surface elsewhere as well. Interestingly, women more than men have abdominal pain whose cause we cannot pinpoint. Often when people come to me suffering from chest or abdominal pains, they are really worried. But we do a full work-up and can't find anything. What they have is *stress*.

Now let me be clear on this point: I'm not saying that most people perceiving pain in a body area without an obvious explanation are just "making it up." You must explore to find out what might be causing it. Pain can be an important wake-up call to the body that something is wrong. Responding to it early, and swiftly, can alleviate the problem before it ever gets serious. As I always remind, it's the body's warning system.

Stress Hormones

Stress also causes your body to release stress hormones.

Hormones such as cortisol and norepinephrine can cause overstimulation of your heart and create palpitations (rapid heartbeat). They also cause higher blood pressure, as these hormones cause vessels to constrict. If you already have the tendency toward high blood pressure on top of these stress hormones, it can shoot your blood pressure very high – over two hundred – and you can have a stroke. Or, if you have unstable plaque inside the arteries, it can cause a major heart attack.

On a less severe note, I often have people show up at my office experiencing palpitations. It's not necessarily something to be immediately alarmed about. This can happen briefly and occasionally with no ill effects. But if it happens for an extended period of time – it can cause you to pass out. While that may sound to some as not particularly serious, think again. Aside from whatever effects it's having on the body, passing out will cause someone to fall, potentially hitting their head or causing other injury. That alone is quite serious. If they happen to be *driving* at the time – there's a whole range of damage that they can do to themselves or others.

Once we check your electrolytes and thyroid, and have also eliminated excessive caffeine as a cause of the palpitations, we will likely address your stress in life. If this turns out to be the source of the problem, most of the time it is cured by having the patient exercise. Among the many benefits of exercise is that it releases endorphins. Endorphins are peptide hormones, which give the person a feeling of well-being. It's very effective! Depression and stress melt away.

There are also those who feel treatments such as acupuncture have the potential to reduce a person's stress. While I have heard anecdotal evidence of this, I'd say it is up to the individual to research and decide for themselves, in the absence of hard scientific proof that I could evaluate.

Being Human Among Humans

As human beings, we constantly interact with each other. That too, at times, can cause stress that it's best to avoid. Not only for your health, but for the relationship itself. Whether it is at work, with family members, or the love of your life – we all have sensitivities. So what can we do?

When stress comes up, you might reframe how you look at things. You might reevaluate what is *truly* important, and how you can resolve problems. A simple example is if you're fighting with your spouse. Sometimes it's best to just walk away. Not to insult them, but so as not to prolong the battle. To ensure no further misunderstanding, it might be good to let them know *why* you're pulling out of the argument. Continuing usually only escalates things; very seldom does it cause anyone to calm down. Once you calm down, you stand a better chance to discover and resolve the issue. However, if stressful arguments repeat continually, you might consider counseling.

Anger is similar to stress in that it releases hormones that stimulate the heart, such that electrical currents to the heart become unstable and make the heart beat faster, creating other problems. It is not good to stay angry.

Ironically, often people are upset with someone about something, and the other person doesn't even know it! We haven't told them. But we think about it, and the more we dwell on it, the more distressed we become. And the more it harms *us*.

So break the pattern. Instead, have a civil conversation with them. *With them.* Not only will this likely reduce the stress, it may well restore the bond, and educate each of you about the other in very valuable ways. All too frequently, our upsets with another are the result of miscommunication or misunderstanding, or simply one or both of us not fully appreciating the needs of the other. Try talking. Ask. Listen. Terrific changes can happen.

In summation, don't settle for *heartache.* Be courageous. Be conscious. Be compassionate.

Let me wrap up this chapter by citing an example of stress causing heart problems...*when you're not even stressing over anything.*

Not the Best Way to Greet the Day

Some people dismiss the following as simply a myth: "There are more heart attacks during the morning hours of five to seven than during any other time of the day."

Naturally, you'd figure this is the last place heart attacks would occur. After all, you're sleeping. You're relaxed. You're not feeling the stress of the day.

But the statement happens to be true.

You release a hormone called cortisol in the early morning. If you recall, cortisol is a stress hormone I described previously. So why is our body releasing it while we're in our comfy sleep-filled bed? The body is designed to help itself get up in the morning by releasing cortisol to help awaken you from your slumber. Very considerate of your body.

However, cortisol can increase your blood pressure significantly if you have the propensity. That increased pressure in the vessels can rupture plaque. If you have unstable plaque in your heart arteries, this cortisol can cause it to rupture and bring on a heart attack. If you have unstable plaque in your neck arteries, that can rupture and cause a stroke.

As you can see, this stress mechanism is primarily chemical. Yes, it can come from worry and upset, or simply your body trying to conduct a natural function (or both – it turns out there is a greater likelihood of heart attacks on *Monday mornings* as people awaken to the stress of returning to work). Aside from reducing stress, your focus should be on improving your cardiovascular health as much as you can. I've already discussed a good diet and exercise. So what is something else you can do for yourself?

Well, it's the topic we've just touched on: sleep.

CHAPTER 25

SLEEP

Don't Take the Lack of It Lying Down

People really do want good health. As a nation, we spend billions of dollars in pursuit of it. We read, we research – hoping to find the secret to its source. Yet many of us ignore one of the most critical factors in our health.

Getting enough sleep.

I believe people are becoming more aware of this. But for a long time, sleep was shunned as not so important. Some would even take pride in their "only needing" five or six hours of sleep to be productive. But studies are showing otherwise. Among the findings: people who sleep less than seven hours a day end up living shorter lives than the general population.

This should serve as an important wake-up call (excuse the pun).

I've had many patients come in with the symptom of fatigue. Why do they see me? Because their tiredness has gotten to a point that they now worry something is wrong with their heart. But the number one cause of fatigue in my experience isn't heart problems – it's lack of sleep. Or interrupted sleep. But that doesn't mean the heart isn't affected. Studies show people getting insufficient sleep over long periods of time will end up having more heart disease.

Yes, you can "get away" with less sleep. But the body needs adequate amounts to recuperate on a daily basis. The benefits of devoting just that little bit of extra time to rest will pay off – big time (again, excuse pun). You'll have more energy for the day, think more clearly, handle stress better, get more done, and generally be happier. And you'll live longer to enjoy it!

Yet too often, we don't make sleep a priority. We trim away at it in order to gain the time to lead the demanding lives we've created. So we get fatigued and less happy. Strangely, some then think the solution to feeling that joy again must be to accomplish *more*.

So...less sleep.

Poor Quality Sleep

For some people, it's not a matter of finding the time to sleep. It's *the sleep itself* that eludes them. They simply can't fall into slumber right away.

Many suffering problems of falling asleep have too much stress in their lives. They're so busy during the day, that when they finally go to bed – it's their first chance to think about everything that is going on – mostly, everything that is causing them stress.

But this is *not* the time to review your day. You can't do anything about it while going to bed anyway. If you must, take some time to review your day before you ever lay down, when you could also write notes to yourself about any actions you may want to take. Once in bed, place all outside issues and thoughts aside, close your eyes and go to sleep. When you put yourself to bed – put your thoughts to bed too.

Something else to keep in mind is that exercise can elevate the hormones (such as endorphins) that relax you, so you'll be less likely to obsess about these things and sleep more easily. If you have a healthy lifestyle and do exercise, your body works so effectively that you sleep much more soundly.

I can't say enough good things about exercise.

Sleep Apnea

Sleep *what??*

Sleep apnea is gaining a lot of attention today, deservedly so. There are estimates that sleep apnea may affect up to 18 million people in the United States and many more worldwide.

People with untreated sleep apnea are fatigued all day. They may think they're sleeping seven or eight hours, but not really. They keep waking up. But they don't know it. They don't become conscious enough to realize that they are awake.

The most common form of this condition is called *obstructive sleep apnea*, in which the throat muscles relax, causing the airway to close. Breathing stops briefly, causing oxygen levels to lower in the blood. Fortunately, the brain recognizes the decrease in the blood oxygen, and sends a signal to awaken the body just enough to reopen the airway and start breathing again. But this whole process can be so subtle that you don't recall waking. It's similar to those who don't realize they snore at night. Usually the sleeping partner is the one that notices the strange sleeping pattern. It's important that they do, as sleep apnea can lead not only to many of the ailments normally associated with too little sleep, including memory loss – it can also contribute to high blood pressure, heart disease and stroke. Recent reports indicate that those with obstructive sleep apnea are at greater risk of having atherosclerosis, as there is more noncalcified plaque in their coronary arteries than those without sleep apnea. In fact, recent studies show those experiencing sleep apnea may have a 30 percent greater risk of dying from heart attacks in their sleep. That is very significant.

Those who suspect they may be suffering from this condition should address it with their cardiologist or general physician. The only way to know with certainty if you have sleep apnea is to be tested, normally in a sleeping diagnostics lab, where they monitor your sleep pattern on a computer. Fortunately, there is treatment. The most typical is using a continuous positive airway pressure device (CPAP) while sleeping. You wear a mask that forces in air to push open the airway so you can breathe and get oxygen into your body. An alternative solution might be the use of a small mouthpiece called a Mandibular Advancement Device, custom fitted by a trained dentist, which readjusts the position of your airway so there is no blockage. In other more severe cases, surgery may be advised.

Notably, recent discoveries have connected other sleeping problems to metabolic syndrome (those risk factors increasing the probability of developing diabetes and cardiovascular disease that I described in Chapter 16). Chronic insomnia and snoring are now thought to be possible indicators of an increased likelihood of developing metabolic syndrome. They may even contribute to causing it. A study showed that difficulty falling asleep increased the probability of metabolic syndrome by 80 percent, while loud snoring (which can accompany sleep apnea) increases the risk by 100 percent (in other words, doubles your chances). Loud snoring was also linked to doubling the odds of developing other metabolic abnormalities.

It should be clear now more than ever, that you need to address chronic sleeping problems, and bring them to the attention of a physician.

CHAPTER 26

SMOKING

Heart Health Risks Go Up in Smoke

Unlike the positive health habits I encourage you to embrace, I want to specifically address one habit that I would strongly avoid.

Of course, it is smoking.

It's common knowledge today that smoking isn't good for your health. As far as heart health, smoking is known to increase LDL cholesterol while lowering HDL. Plus, it elevates levels of triglycerides somewhat. It also promotes atherosclerosis (plaque formation) in the arteries' inner lining and increases the risk of forming blood clots. Smoking can also significantly accelerate peripheral arterial disease (PAD) – atherosclerosis in the arteries outside of the heart that go to the periphery – including those to the kidneys, the stomach, and legs. As said previously, smokers are four times as likely to contract PAD as nonsmokers.

Curiously, it's not entirely clear how smoking does all this. There's likely a tie-in to its negative impact on cholesterol levels. It might also involve the nicotine constricting blood vessels. Or the carbon monoxide damaging vessels' inner lining. Or the diminishment of the oxygen going through the blood, which becomes an even bigger issue as the heart needs to circulate *more* oxygen to offset smoking's other negative effects. There are about 4,000 chemicals in cigarettes and we still don't know all the effects they might have on a body.

Whatever the cause, it's believed that men smoking even just 20 cigarettes a day (not a lot for many smokers), are *three times* more likely to have a heart attack than those who've never smoked. Statistics for women are even more startling: female smokers of 20 cigarettes daily are *six times* more likely to suffer a heart attack.

You'd think these numbers alone would be enough to convince people to stop. Unfortunately, it is very difficult for smokers to give up their habit. Smoking is addictive, but smokers can also live in a certain denial. Some like to cite that "everyone knows" of somebody who smoked and drank and lived to a ripe old age.

Yet I've noticed something in my practice that is pretty telling. I see a wide variety of patients in many age groups. Of all the patients that I have over 80 – only one or two still smoke. *Almost every single one* of my patients living past 80, have never smoked in the past or quit smoking – and quit at least 10 or 20 years prior – not just a year or two earlier. That's a very clear marker in my patient population of the effects of smoking. Other patients who continued to be smokers have already passed away from one ailment or another, be it heart attack, stroke, lung disease or cancer.

Notably, if one of my smoking patients experiences an event – a heart attack, stroke, or ends up getting a stent in the heart – then they stop smoking. Suddenly they find the will power and commitment. Perhaps until that point – it's too "inconvenient" to believe what they're told. But once something happens, they correlate that event to the smoking, and fear convinces them to stop.

Of course, it would be far better if they take that step *before* they have a heart attack.

CHAPTER 27

SYMPTOMS OF HEART DISEASE
Paying Attention

By this time, I hope you are grasping the big role you play in your heart health. I've addressed creating positive health habits with a good diet, plentiful exercise, reduction of stress, adequate sleep, and elimination of smoking.

So aside from doing all this – should you see a cardiologist?

If you have *no* risk factors (high blood pressure, cholesterol, family history, diabetes, smoking), and have *no* symptoms, then you really don't need to see a cardiologist. Just keep up your routine testing with your physician.

But if you *are* having symptoms – *pay attention*.

Your body possesses a terrific feedback system. It can give clues that something is going on – if you know what to look for. The catchphrase that heart disease is "the silent killer," is largely true because people don't know how to "listen." It is a tragic fact that for 50 percent of those people who have heart attacks – the first sign of heart disease they recognize is a heart attack with sudden death.

Obviously, this is not the way you want to learn that you have a coronary condition.

While some patients might become upset when there is a signal indicating they may have a problem, my attitude is *thank goodness we got the warning!* That way we can address the problem before it becomes too serious.

So what are these warning signs? They vary somewhat, depending on the particular heart disease causing them. But they are all good indicators.

Coronary Disease

With coronary disease or arterial blockages that can lead to heart attacks, typical symptoms can include chest pressure when exerting yourself. The feeling is like an elephant sitting on the chest, and can radiate to the left shoulder or left arm. It may be accompanied with nausea or sweating. Some people are aware of these as indicators of a heart attack, but you don't need to be experiencing a heart attack for these to occur. A blockage somewhere is obstructing the free-flow of your blood, such that the exertion's demand on the heart is too much for the amount of blood and oxygen it's receiving. Typically, you might be going up stairs and feel that pressure on your chest. Then you stop and it goes away. You start up the stairs again, it will come back. Another classic example is while someone mows their lawn. They feel the pressure. Then they stop and it goes away. They start up again and it returns. That's a definite warning sign. We would call these typical angina symptoms.

There can also be *atypical* symptoms. These are more common in women and diabetic patients. It often consists of diffuse sweating, as opposed to chest pressure. Or they have shortness of breath with no chest pressure. Or they can feel more fatigued than usual when they do any activity (more about women's symptoms in Chapter 33). These are atypical symptoms that may arise from blockages in the arteries.

Congestive Heart Failure

Congestive heart failure also presents certain warning signs.

Different causes can lead to heart failure. It might be valve disease caused by a virus. Occasionally it is drug-induced. Sometimes it occurs after a heart attack when your heart becomes weakened. If you have heart failure, you generally experience shortness of breath from exertion (similar to coronary disease). Secondly, you also experience shortness of breath when you lie down. When you sit up – the shortness of breath gets better. Or your legs swell more than is normal. You might also feel your heart going a little fast, as it has to compensate for being weak. Sometimes you simply feel fatigued.

PAD

Unfortunately, many of those with peripheral arterial disease show no outward symptoms. For those that do, warning signs most often are pain when walking (which stops upon rest), or cramps or numbness in your legs, or even discoloration of skin or sores on the legs. But again, one must realize that even if these symptoms are confined primarily to the legs, when one has atherosclerosis in one area, it's likely to be in other vessels in the body as well.

Valve Disease

Chest pains can accompany valve disease, as the heart has to work harder. The next likely indicator would be passing out. The third progressive symptom would be heart failure. If you have leaky valve or have a mitral valve – it's shortness of breath and fatigue.

Being Aware

As you can see, many of the symptoms are similar across different diseases, though the origins are different. In summary, the telltale symptoms you might look for are:

- Chest pressure during exertion that may radiate to the left shoulder or arm, possibly accompanied by nausea or sweating
- Chest pressure during exertion (as in going up stairs), stops when you stop, then resumes when exerting again
- Shortness of breath when exerting
- Shortness of breath when you lie down that improves when you sit up
- More fatigued than usual
- Swelling in the legs
- Diffuse sweating
- Any of these accompanied by a rapid heartbeat
- Passing out

Heart Attack

Of course, we are hoping to recognize symptoms of heart disease early enough so that we never experience a heart attack. But if one should happen, you should know what to look for.

There are classical signs and there are atypical signs. The classical sign is chest pain that feels like pressure, comes on with exertion, lasts at least a minute or longer, and occurs in the area beneath the sternum. It can also radiate to the left arm. Atypical signs can be anything from fatigue and tiredness to diffuse sweating.

So how to know if you should be worried? In a nutshell, if you have a history of heart attacks or blockages, or of diabetes, smoking, high blood pressure, or are of an older age – then you should consider any symptom as potentially serious. See your doctor as soon as possible, or if serious enough, call 911. Keep in mind to always chew a *full-strength* aspirin immediately at the onset of chest pain. I recommend chewing, as it absorbs much faster into your system. This can significantly reduce the chance of dying from heart attack.

Again, the focus is on noticing heart disease symptoms early on and successfully correcting the cause before there's ever a heart attack or stroke. Fortunately, this is something we are commonly able to do.

A Living Example

A young bank security guard, who reported feeling unusually short of breath while recently being active, was referred to me. The shortness of breath appeared suddenly and had already lasted a few days without getting any better. The only other symptom he had was a somewhat rapid heartbeat.

Two things could be going on in this young man. Either he has a weak heart, or he had a large blood clot in his lungs affecting his heart. I immediately had my echo technician do an ultrasound of the heart (echocardiogram). It showed the right chambers of the heart to be extremely dilated. That meant there was a resistance to blood pumping from the right side of the heart to the lungs. That is usually caused by a large blood clot sitting in the lungs, which comes from the leg.

Right away, I sent him to get a CAT scan. It showed a huge blood clot in his lungs. If I hadn't tested him and had simply sent him home, he would have died in his bed that night. Instead, I treated him with blood thinners and he's doing very well. I took an assertive approach to uncover what was occurring and it paid off. Being able to make a quick diagnosis and intervene quickly, leading to helping a young person with all his life still ahead of him, is a very satisfying feeling that makes me forget all those sleepless nights when we doctors wake up to assist our patients.

Your Simple Job

Part of a good cardiologist's responsibility is to know how aggressively to pursue testing and treatment, given the patient's symptoms, risk factors, general health history, etc.

Your job is much simpler: whether you get some major or minor symptoms of a heart issue – *pay attention*. Do not ignore this warning gift. Not everyone is fortunate enough to experience or recognize them. Be grateful. Be proactive.

And tell your doctor.

CHAPTER 28

THE CARDIOLOGIST'S OFFICE

Unveiling the Mystery

Now that you have a good understanding of basic heart health, I want you to become comfortable with what a typical visit might be like to your cardiologist. My intention is not only to further educate, but also to remove the mystery and perhaps accompanying fears.

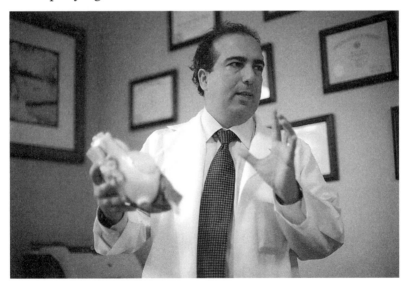

Contrary to what you might think, patients often come to me that don't have any serious health issues. Commonly, they are simply middle-aged with at least one other risk factor. They might have high cholesterol, high blood pressure, or their father had a heart attack at a young age. They have no other symptoms and seem to be doing just fine. They come to make sure there are no unknown conditions and to improve their heart health, while preventing any problems from forming.

On the other hand, I will also see patients who've noticed some significant symptom, which they think might be connected to heart disease.

In either case, patients may have some apprehension about seeing a cardiologist. They worry the visit may reveal some bad news. When someone new comes in for an initial visit, before they've gotten to know me, they are often nervous. In fact, there's almost always what is commonly called "white coat hypertension." That means they're so anxious coming to the doctor (who wears a white coat), that their blood pressure is highly elevated. Yet at home, it may be normal.

Knowing all this guides how I work with my patients. I'm very compassionate when speaking with them. If they are coming in after some symptom has presented itself, there is a good chance I'm going to find some issue. I try to give them a better perspective, if I must tell them news they might not want to hear. I point out that at least we found the problem and thank goodness we discovered it. If they had waited longer, there might have been a major heart attack. So let's deal with it now.

So let me explain how a visit to your cardiologist would likely unfold, and help remove a bit of the anxiety.

Family History

One of the first criteria I explore with patients is whether there is a strong history of heart disease in the family. We define this as if there are close female relatives who died from heart ailments before the age of 65, or men before 55. If either of those is the case, that is considered a "positive family history."

But family heart disease doesn't only mean someone has died from the illness. Someone having a heart attack or a bypass or a stent for a blockage are all considered a positive family history. Why is this important? Because research has found that heart disease is often genetic. For instance, if one of your parents had high blood pressure, there is genetic likelihood that you're more likely to have it as well.

Maybe it's not the news you wanted to hear, but it is something you want to know. For while there's nothing you can do to evade genetics, you can offset the genetic tendency by exercising, losing weight and not taking too many anti-inflammatory medications such as Motrin, that can affect blood pressure. So being aware of family history is important, and you should learn as many details about your parents' history as you can. Now, it is possible to lose weight, improve eating and exercise habits, and still have high blood pressure. But all of those actions can still help.

I have some young patients with high blood pressure, and when they exercise and lose weight – their blood pressure drops. It may remain higher than we'd like, but down it goes. Then medication helps reduce it further. So it's important to know your family history even while you're relatively young. It used to be that the onset of high blood pressure didn't occur until later in life. But now it's becoming more prevalent at young ages. This is largely due to the epidemic of obesity that we're experiencing. Obesity not only brings on diabetes, but also increases the risk of hypertension.

Sometimes You Get Lucky

It should be noted that while a family history of heart disease doesn't work in your favor, some people actually have a "genetic blueprint" for *not* having cardiovascular disease. They have hereditary protection. These people might smoke, eat poorly and seldom exercise – and never develop blockages. That's why it's never wise for someone who doesn't want to give up a vice or bad health habit to cite "Uncle Joe" who smoked two packs every day of his life and lived to be 95. Though rather rare, some "Uncle Joes" have this unique genetic make-up that protects them. But don't simply expect that you can duplicate their behavior and not create heart disease in yourself.

A dramatic form of this genetic protection is a special type of gene that exists in an extended family residing in a village near Milan, Italy. The gene they share significantly *raises* their good cholesterol. Named "A-1 Milano," it actually can *get rid* of fat-caused plaque. The result is these people hardly have any blockages whatsoever! Lucky for them – and for us. From studying the genes of these people, scientists have developed new medications. So when people come in with heart attacks, not only can we give blood thinners, it may be possible to inject them with a medication with byproducts of these good genes that can clean up these fats right away (so far, they are still experimental and not yet FDA approved).

Like I said, research continues on and on.

Risk Factors

Aside from learning their family history, I also explore whether my patients possess any of the other known risk factors for coronary disease and heart attacks. These would include:

- hypertension
- cholesterol levels
- their age
- stress levels
- sedentary lifestyle
- obesity
- diabetes
- smoking
- type-A personality

This information is essential in my evaluating the likelihood of their having some issue and its severity. It also factors into how aggressive I should be if I find some condition – whether we can keep an eye on the issue as we begin medication or treatment, or if I need to admit them to the hospital right away.

Blood Tests

One of the primary methods of testing is through blood work. The most basic is testing for cholesterol. Generally, that's the blood test most primary care physicians perform in regards to heart heath. As described earlier in my chapter focused on cholesterol, I always suggest going beyond the most basic cholesterol panels to do the VAP test.

However, the cardiologist is likely to perform additional testing.

Homocysteine

Homocysteine is an amino acid and an important building block for protein. However, a very high level of homocysteine in someone's blood can be a contributor to – and an indicator for – having higher occurrences of coronary disease.

The treatment for too much homocysteine is basically folic acid, a B-vitamin supplement – along with vitamins B-6 and B-12. They help break down the homocysteine so there's less in your system. But there is a controversy attached to this today. While doctors have long strived to lower homocysteine levels, recent studies are showing that even if you treat it successfully, you really don't change the likelihood of coronary disease. So doctors generally have stopped treating homocysteine levels. They still may *test for it as an indicator*, but most don't try to reduce it.

Fibrinogen

Fibrinogen is a protein made by the liver, which gets activated into becoming fibrin, which is basically a clot. So fibrinogen is seen as a precursor to clot formation.

As already described, heart attacks and strokes occur when you have plaque in the arteries that either erodes (into the artery lining) or ruptures. In either case, you can get blood clot formation and then a stroke or heart attack. Therefore, the conclusion is those people with much more fibrinogen are at higher risks.

But at present, there is no medication to lower fibrinogen. It again is simply seen as a warning sign.

CRP

C-reactive protein is a protein in the blood. It can also provide a clue to the likelihood of heart disease, as levels of CRP rise in response to inflammation.

Understand that when you have blockages in the arteries, it is an inflammatory state. Therefore, the CRP serves as a good marker of the amount of blockages all over your body. If measurements show it to be less than one, that's normal. One through three is borderline, and above three is abnormal.

In general, we test twice, separated by a couple of weeks, and take the average. That is because the flu or some other infections can also raise the CRP level. We also take into account that people who have a chronic inflammatory disorder, such as an immune disease like rheumatoid arthritis, will already have an elevated level. That's why if the test result is more than 10, we discount it, because it must be sourcing from some inflammatory disease rather than from arteries.

CHAPTER 29

TECHNOLOGY ON OUR SIDE

Testing Today for Heart Health

In addition to the already described blood work, there is a wide variety of sophisticated testing available to cardiologists today that can precisely reveal the otherwise hidden details of your heart health.

EKG

First, let me address one of the more common tests that has been around for some time. An electrocardiogram, often called an EKG, measures changes in the electrical activity of your heart. Electrodes are attached via wires onto your chest that link back to the EKG machine.

The machine not only calculates how fast your heart is beating, but also shows your heartbeat's rhythm, plus the strength and timing of the electrical signals in your heart. It can reveal an arrhythmia, whether you've had or are currently experiencing a heart attack, or have heart failure.

Echocardiogram

Another test that's long been available is an echocardiogram. It employs sound waves to actually recreate a moving image of the heart. This representation offers a more detailed picture than a normal X-ray, but requires no radiation

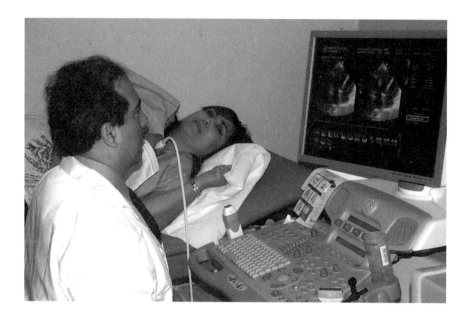

exposure. A device called a transducer is placed on your breast-bone and generates high-frequency sound waves. It picks up the echoes (hence its name) of these sound waves as electrical impulses, transforming them into a moving image of the heart. An echocardiogram permits doctors to view the heart and its structure *as it beats*.

Of course, testing for heart health isn't limited to tests just on the heart. As you hopefully understand by now, heart health very much involves your *vascular system* as well.

CIMT

CIMT stand for Carotid Intima Media Thickness (you can see why we use the abbreviation). One of cardiology's newer tests, it's a consequence of the fairly recent discovery that if we measure the thickening of the inside lining of the carotid artery, and compare it to the average thickness for the normal population, we can actually predict your chances of having a heart attack or stroke in the future. A relatively inexpensive test, the CIMT scan is absolutely painless. It employs ultrasound digital technology and software, and only requires five to ten minutes to perform.

Research has revealed a 90 percent probability between finding atherosclerosis in the carotid artery and the disease being elsewhere in the body. In a way, CIMT tests give an approximation of the "age" of your blood vessels compared to your real age.

Again, some people might say, "Don't give me that test! I don't want to know." Then again, if they *did* know, we'd have a better sense how aggressive we need to be in improving their heart health. That is a *good* thing.

My neighbor, a man I waved to most every day, was seemingly in good health at 47. He came to my office with only borderline high blood pressure, but with high cholesterol. Not wanting to take pills, he would make excuses like, "If I take these cholesterol medications, I can't sleep." So he was taking *half of a half* of the lowest dose of the medication. His cholesterol numbers reflected this. They still looked pretty bad.

I informed him that the medication has nothing to do with sleep. He couldn't use that as an excuse for not taking his medicine.

But he wasn't budging. I ended up doing a CIMT on him. A simple test, it uses ultrasound to noninvasively measure the thickness of the inside lining of the carotid artery. Indeed, the results turned out higher than they should be for someone his age. I explained that this suggested his risk of heart attack or stroke was much greater than for other people. I also told him that while exercise would help, it wouldn't solve his problem. I emphasized again that his medication doesn't cause problems with sleep and that he needed to be more aggressive in taking it, or he likely could develop blockages and have a heart attack. "And then what will your kids do for a father?"

That he listened to.

I wasn't trying to scare him (okay, maybe a little), but I wanted him to fully grasp the situation. This CIMT test is pretty definitive in predicting serious risks.

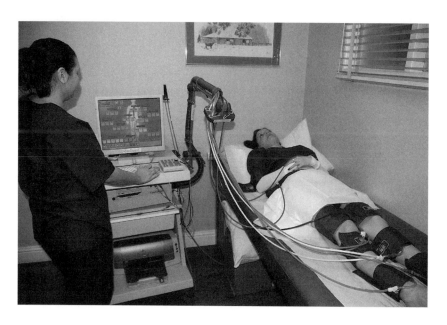

Testing for PAD

If you recall, peripheral arterial disease (PAD) is when plaque has built-up in the arteries traveling to your "periphery" – the outer regions of your body. That includes those that carry blood to your head, your limbs, and organs. This can lead to atherosclerosis, hardening the plaque, and narrowing the arteries – reducing blood flow to those areas.

While this may not be noticeable to someone, I have described that symptoms can often show up in your legs, where blocked blood flow causes numbness and/or pain. If you experience pain in your legs when you climb stairs or just walk, you should talk with your doctor. Sometimes people ignore this advice, believing their leg pain is simply a symptom that comes along with getting older. But it might be due to PAD, which is why you consult your physician.

If we suspect a patient has peripheral arterial disease, we first diagnose by comparing blood pressure in the legs to that in the arms, using an ABI (ankle-brachial) test.

That helps demonstrate the quality of your blood flow, and is a surprisingly good indicator not only of plaque buildup in the leg arteries, but also a good determinant of buildup in the whole cardiovascular system. Normal ankle pressure should be at least 90 percent as high as in the arm. But if there is serious atherosclerosis, its narrowing will reduce it to possibly less than half.

Cardiovascular Profiler (CVP)

Sometimes my patients ask, "If I correct the behaviors that caused the damage to my arteries' inner linings – can the damage be reversed?"

I reply, "To a great extent, poor endothelium function is reversible, at least at the early initial levels."

That's when they get excited, and a little skeptical. "Really?"

"Yes. In fact, not only can you reverse the damage – I can *prove* it to you."

I inform them of a machine in my office called a Cardiovascular Profiler, or CVP. I explain that this device evaluates the endothelium function. Secondarily, it measures elasticity of the vessels. As previously mentioned, the first thing creating atherosclerosis is that the endothelium function goes bad and you develop blockages. (Diabetics, by the nature of their microvascular disease, almost always have abnormal endothelium function.)

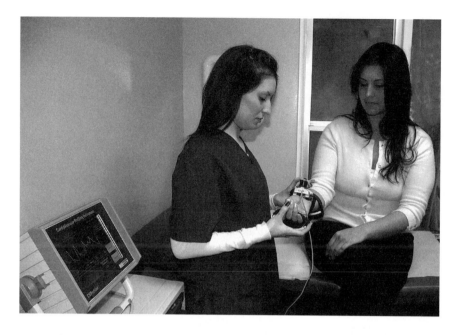

This test uses an ultrasound probe placed over the radial artery of the arm, and only takes five minutes.

It yields a result that I can compare to that which a healthy patient should have for their age and gender. This helps guide my therapy for the patient. If the results are not good, I may encourage that you exercise, lower your weight, lower your blood pressure and your cholesterol (possibly aided by medication). Then I see you in a few months and we do this test again. If you've complied with some or all of my suggestions, the results will prove your arteries are indeed becoming healthier. It is a terrific tool to motivate patients to stick with new healthier regimens for themselves. All too often, patients are advised to change health habits with the promise of various life-protecting benefits. But they don't stick with it since they can't see the results (you can't "see" an absence of a heart attack). With this machine, I can show them tangible proof that what they're doing is benefiting their lives.

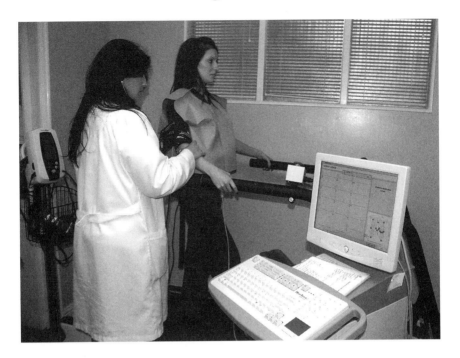

Microvolt T-Wave Alternans (MTWA)

Another excellent tool, this device yields results as good as if giving a full invasive EP evaluation, to see if there is an arrhythmia causing someone to have syncope (a neurological condition where someone feels lightheaded, dizzy, and may pass out).

Instead of an electrophysiologist inserting a probe through a leg vein up to the heart to map where there may be electrical shortages, the MTWA uses a simple treadmill test. During this test, a special computer analyzes an electrocardiogram at the microvolt level that is known to cause arrhythmias.

This MTWA allows us to determine if the patient is at high risk of arrhythmias leading to sudden death, and that I need to implant an automatic defibrillator in the patient to solve the problem (as will be described in Chapter 31, a defibrillator is a device that sends a therapeutic dose of electrical current into a person's body to normalize heart function in certain life-threatening situations).

BioZ Impedance Cardiography (ICG)

Without my even needing to go inside a blood vessel in the body, this test gives me the hemodynamics of the cardiovascular system. It involves hooking up some special electrodes to the patient's body.

It's often performed for someone experiencing shortness of breath, as it reveals if there is fluid in the lungs, and/or if systemic vascular resistance in the vessel is causing the problem. I also may give this test to someone on multiple blood pressure drugs, allowing me to fine tune their medications, based on objective findings rather than estimations.

As example, I did a BioZ test on a patient with heart failure, who was experiencing low blood pressure and shortness of breath. The results showed the shortness of breath was due to his systemic vascular resistance being elevated. I gave him a medication that normally would drop blood pressure (something I *didn't* want to occur), but with this medication reducing the vascular resistance, the heart muscle was able to pump more effectively, and at the same time be better able to maintain blood pressure. I could measure all this on the machine. The shortness of breath then went away because the heart wasn't backing pressure up to the lungs.

Electron Beam Computerized Tomography (EBCT)

An Ultrafast CAT scan of the chest, the EBCT reports a "calcium score," which is a good predictor of heart disease developing in a patient's future. A particularly high score can also tell us there's a strong chance of a significant blockage already present.

In coronary artery disease, the plaque that causes blockages is composed somewhat of calcium. The EBCT can detect this calcium in the arteries that may lead to creating blockages.

Because it is so sensitive, this test is especially useful for younger patients at risk for developing coronary disease, who wouldn't yet have large amounts of calcium in their arteries. Test results can show if a patient is likely to develop serious coronary disease. (Older patients probably already have some significant buildup of calcium, so this test isn't quite as useful of a predictor for them).

There is some controversy about this procedure, however, as it does expose the patient to additional radiation. A doctor should be judicious in deciding when to use it, taking into account past radiation exposures of the patient.

CHAPTER 30

MORE AGGRESSIVE DIAGNOSTICS
Invasive and Noninvasive Testing

As I indicated before, along with those simply wanting to learn if they're at risk of heart disease, many patients come to my office for the first time presenting symptoms. They're among the many that wait until they think something is wrong before consulting a doctor. They might come in with chest pains, shortness of breath, diffuse sweating, or any of the other signs already described.

Based on their family history and other risk factors, I access the chances of their having heart disease. If they have borderline risk, I'll do some of the noninvasive tests just described: the blood work, carotid intima media thickness (CIMT), cardiovascular profiler (CVP), or electron beam computer tomography (EBCT).

But if I feel they have more than an intermediate risk – such as if they're diabetic, a smoker, or older – and the symptoms they're presenting indicate a good chance of a blockage, more aggressive testing is necessary.

It is ideal to take all information into account to formulate a plan, rather than taking a cookbook approach where one "recipe" fits all. This alludes to an important difference between doctors. Some are more like technicians. They simply anyone shows a particular symptom, then there's a response. But the human body is more complex than ~~~ ~~ ~~diagnosed through some universal checklist. We must take into account the whole spectrum of the patient's history, all the risk factors, as well as their current condition and EKG test before making a decision.

Treadmill Test

If there is a probable chance they have blockages, the simplest test to perform is the exercise treadmill test, also called a stress test.

A patient's blood pressure and heart rate are monitored, along with EKG testing, as the patient moves through a series of short (three minute) sequences of walking/running on a treadmill, as the speed and angle are increased. This test can be administered only to patients who have a normal EKG when at rest. The treadmill test can detect blockages accurately up to about 70 percent of cases. But that also means that even if the test turns out normal, there's still a 30 percent chance of an undetected blockage.

So based on the patient and the results of this test, we make a decision whether we need to study further in order to raise the accuracy up to 85 or 90 percent. We do that by adding imaging to this stress test, likely with an echocardiogram done in the office. Images are taken via ultrasound when the patient is at rest, and immediately after completing the treadmill test.

This test is definitely a step up in its ability to detect, and is very good if you have a lot of blockages. The only problem with a stress echocardiogram is that it is not very good at picking up a singular vessel blockage in the heart arteries, or if the blockages are just borderline.

CT Angiogram (CTA)

The next level of non-invasive testing is a fairly new approach – a CT angiogram. (They can now even use a PET scan or a cardiac MRI to perform similar tests). These detect even better than any of the previous noninvasive techniques. Accurate and sensitive, they pick up microvascular blockages at over 95 percent accuracy.

The pros of the CT angiogram are that it is noninvasive and less risky to the patient. The cons are that it doses the patient with substantial radiation, plus you're still having a contrast injected into your blood to enhance the visuals, which could damage kidneys if they are already compromised.

So my criteria for having a patient get a CT angiogram is they must have normal kidney function, and haven't had too many CT and X-rays in the past. Then having a CT angiogram once or twice in a lifetime is okay.

Nuclear Imaging Evaluation

Another step above what has been described so far is a Nuclear Imaging Evaluation (Myocardial Perfusion Imaging). A radioactive isotope is injected into a vein, allowing us to measure the blood flow to your heart muscle at rest or while on a treadmill.

This imaging is actually done two times – once under resting conditions, and again under stress, such as exercise. The idea is that if the demand for oxygen goes up with stress such as exercise, and the supply is not met because of a blockage in the artery, then there will be less radioisotope uptake by the heart muscle. When this is compared to the resting image, it helps us detect the amount of blockage and the location. This test normally carries 90 percent accuracy in detecting blockages in the heart arteries.

Appropriate Testing

I don't bring up all these various forms of testing because I want you to memorize them. But I do want you to appreciate the vast selection of testing available today. We are fortunate. As said before, cardiology has truly advanced, and you should seek out a doctor who is at the forefront of this knowledge and technology. But be clear on one thing: it's not that you necessarily should get many or even some of these tests. It's not about cardiologists performing too many tests. Not at all. Doctors should give the appropriate testing for the appropriate patients at the appropriate times. The reasons for giving tests should be evidence based.

Yet it should also be appreciated that today, these noninvasive tests, whether separately or together, get results close to that long-desired 100 percent accuracy – determining whether there are blockages, and the condition of our blood vessels.

Invasive Testing: The Angiogram – Improved

The longtime "gold star" of all tests to see if there are blockages causing a patient's symptoms is the coronary angiogram. This procedure not only can diagnose – it can also *correct* the problem.

This procedure is done in a hospital, where a small plastic tube called a catheter is inserted through the large femoral artery in the patient's thigh, up nearly to the heart. Through this tube, a special dye is injected as an X-ray observes its movement – to see in real time if there are any blockages interfering with its flow through coronary arteries.

Having been around awhile, it's now been enhanced – with stents.

Correcting with Stents

As I said, this testing protocol is unusual in that the procedure can also be used to correct the problem, by opening up a blockage in an artery.

In the old days, we had "balloon angioplasty." A tiny balloon at the end of a catheter was inserted up the artery to the point of the blockage, where it would be inflated. That would crush the blockage into the periphery of the artery and open up the blood flow. But there was a problem with this approach. You could still have "rebound reflex" that might cause a tear in the artery and make it suddenly shut down. But it was the best procedure we had.

Until we developed stenting.

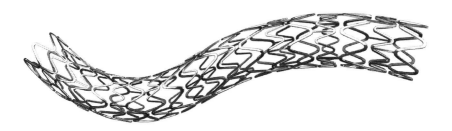

Image provided courtesy of Boston Scientific. © 2011 Boston Scientific Corporation or its affiliates. All rights reserved

A stent is a small stainless steel tube placed in a coronary artery to keep the vessel open and blood flowing.

Inserting a stent is done fairly similarly to the balloon angioplasty. A tiny balloon is still slipped into the artery pathway, but there's also a stainless steel tube that sits around the balloon. When both are inserted up to the point of a blockage, the balloon inflates to open up the artery – which also causes the stent to spring open into its full position. The cylindrical stent prevents any rebound and potential tear from occurring. Then the balloon is deflated and withdrawn, but the now open stent remains – to ensure that the artery stays open and clear. Even if there is a small tear, the stent allows it to heal. This procedure is so successful that even if a blockage is up to 99 percent closed, most of the time we can get the balloon and stent in there. They're wrapped very tightly, until you balloon it in and the stent springs open.

This new technique offered great improvement in opening blockages. Patients fared much better. But then something happened. It is odd, but sometimes when a new technology solves one problem, another comes with it that must be resolved as well.

In this case, there was a problem with using the stents. It was realized that when a damaged artery would heal around the stent, it sometimes would form scar tissue, usually within the first three months (some people form more scar tissue than others, such as diabetics). Scar formation can eventually lead to another blockage. These people would then often have to come back to redo the procedure.

Fortunately, we solved the problem. We came up with "medicated stents" (also called "drug-eluting stents" or DES). These stents slowly release a drug over two to three months that prevents this scar formation. So using these new stents, we got rid of the scarring.

But then, maybe you guessed it...we had a *new* problem.

Turned out that the medicated stent was *so good* at preventing scar formation, that sometimes part of the stent was left exposed because the artery wouldn't grow any tissue around it at all. But we want the stent to become part of the arterial wall with a small lining growing over it, in effect "becoming" part of the body. If that doesn't happen and a portion of the stent remains exposed, it can form sudden blood clots as it is "seen" as a foreign body to your system. That's serious. You can have a major heart attack.

So, how do we deal with this?

When originally implanting unmedicated stents (which may also be referred to as "bare-metal stents"), we routinely put patients on blood thinners for two to three months to keep blockages from forming. But we found these newer medicated stents can take up to six months to a year to integrate into the artery wall. So now it's recommended that all doctors have those patients on blood thinners for a year to be safe, followed by taking aspirin, which acts as a blood thinner to ensure no blood clots form later. So we now have protocols to solve the inherent problems associated with these stents, and today they are very effective in helping patients.

As you might imagine, these stents are fairly expensive. Plus you may need more than one in a procedure. But if they can ensure your health, as well as prevent the need for another procedure – believe me, they are well worth it.

Bypass Surgery

I should mention that as wonderful as stenting is, if a patient has certain blockages and medical conditions (such as blockages in the three main arteries, plus a weakened heart, and is diabetic), a patient may benefit more from a bypass surgery rather than from stents, as there is a better survival rate.

Coronary artery bypass surgery has been performed since the 1960s. The aorta is the main artery coming from the heart, which in turn connects to various coronary arteries that flow blood to the rest of the body. If there is a significant blockage in this aorta that is not suitable for stenting, a cardiovascular surgeon takes a portion of a vein from the patient's leg. The surgeon attaches one end of this vein into the aorta, while the other end of the vein is then grafted into a coronary artery *on the other side* of the blockage – thereby *bypassing* the blockage. In a way, it is creating a "bridge" over which blood can flow.

While more of a major surgery than stenting, bypass surgery is very straightforward, has been performed successfully for years, and saves lives when needed.

CHAPTER 31

THE DEFIBRILLATOR

Shocking Health

When correcting for heart disease, the first avenue I like to pursue is using medications. They are less invasive than any surgery, less risky, and easier on the patient. I will address the remarkable variety of medications that have been developed for cardiology today in Chapters 37 through 42.

In addition to medication, there is the range of surgeries that can be used in serious cases. Stenting and angioplasty are forms of this. So are more invasive procedures, such as bypass and valve surgeries. Those I leave up to surgeons who specialize in those more dramatic interventions. Of course, a cardiologist's wish is to avoid surgery whenever possible, through medication or other treatments.

Cardiologists do install the pacemakers that I described in Chapter 12, as well as perform angioplasty and stenting. There's also another surgical procedure cardiologists perform, using a fantastic state-of-the-art device that saves lives.

On Automatic: the Internal Cardiac Defibrillator

There's a term in cardiology called cardiomyopathy. It means the heart's ability to squeeze out the blood (ejection fraction) has fallen below 35 percent. Normal would be 60 percent. Ejection fraction is one of the best predictors of someone's longevity. Studies in recent years have shown that patients with ejection fraction of less than 35 percent are at high risk of tachycardic arrhythmias or sudden cardiac death.

People may develop this heart muscle dysfunction for various reasons. A heart attack can leave the muscle weak. Or perhaps a valve malfunction wasn't treated at the proper time. It might be due to high blood pressure that hasn't been under control for many years. Occasionally, a virus or bacteria can cause it. Sometimes we simply don't know the cause (and yes, we have a word for that too: idiopathic).

With cardiomyopathy, basically the chamber of the heart dilates (opens up) and the ability to squeeze lessens. We use an echocardiogram to determine the strength of the squeeze of the heart. If it is too weak, the recommendation is they get an Automatic Internal Cardiac Defibrillator (AICD).

As mentioned earlier, a defibrillator sends a therapeutic dose of electrical current into a person's body to normalize heart function in various life-threatening situations. They're traditionally the "crash carts" on TV hospital shows where paddles are placed on a person's chest, someone shouts "clear," and the patient's body shakes as their heart is "shocked" back into beating correctly. It helps to be in the hospital when you need one, or have a paramedic only minutes away. But that's not always the case. Plus, you may have heard stories of people suddenly dying in their bed while asleep. If related to the heart, it's mostly due to an arrhythmia. People with arrhythmias lasting a long time don't get blood flow to the brain. They die. Unless someone shocks them out of it right away.

That's why an AICD is so extraordinary. It's different from a normal defibrillator in two primary ways:

- it is automatic
- it is implanted inside a person's body

How it works is pretty interesting. This defibrillator is a smart generator that diagnoses. As soon as it detects a person's heart rate rise to a certain level, for example 160 or 170, it immediately can identify the type of arrhythmia and tries to rapidly pace the heart out of it. If that doesn't work within a minute or two, then it shocks the heart.

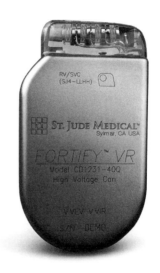

Not only that, these units are so advanced, they can also send a signal to the company and the doctor that this event is occurring! Then an ambulance is called to the house. The device sends this information through a "docking station" in the home connected to the phone line. The docking station is even small enough that it can be taken along whenever the person travels and connected to another landline. There are also versions now that can dock with your cell phone to send an alert to your doctor.

This technology was very notable at the time it first appeared, such that when I implanted my first one, a story appeared in the local newspaper as it was the first done in this part of California. Now I implant these all the time. They absolutely save lives.

CHAPTER 32

HUMAN SIDE OF HEART HEALTH
Treating Patients with Patience

I'm hoping you are feeling a bit more assured, now that you're acquainted with a vast variety of tests and solutions available through a cardiologist. For most, it is a welcome relief to better understand heart health.

Of course, cardiologists aren't just treating symptoms and conditions. Good ones are treating the *whole* patient. Doctors are aware of the anxieties that patients may bring to the office, along with their symptoms and heart history. That's why a good approach is to be compassionate, while educating patients, explaining their particular options, and exploring the best treatment for each individual.

Still, whenever I must deliver not-so-great news, some patients react much as anyone might to something they don't like. It's the classic four stages. First they deny. Then they get angry (not at me, but very possibly at God or whoever). Then they try to negotiate (often with God, promising "If you help me, I'll behave better," etc). Let's Make a Deal time.

Then finally, they accept. I experience all these stages with them in my office. Sometimes within a matter of minutes. I've also had patients informed of their condition who suddenly break into tears. Or some adamant about trying other avenues before any kind of surgery. Still others want it all taken care of right away. I've literally had people respond, "Can we do the surgery this afternoon?"

Fortunately, our first approach to solving most cardiac issues is through medication. In fact, as I'll explain in more detail later in my chapters on drugs, I am an interventional cardiologist. I prefer to intervene before surgery is required. But I am also a scientist. I go by what research has taught us. If someone's condition isn't a type that can be helped by medication, then I will recommend surgery. I must for the patient's well-being.

We always weigh benefits versus risk. But if your noninvasive testing showed significant areas at risk because they're not getting enough oxygen, I'd explain that even if we gave you medication, the danger would remain high. I would recommend that we schedule hospital time to go in and explore in the artery to find out exactly what is going on.

High Degree of Confidence

Ultimately, the patient may need to have surgery. But having performed so many successfully over time, I have a realistically high degree of confidence where I can be successful. Yet all this is new to the patient. They mostly have uncertainty and apprehension, and as a result, often a hesitancy to take the appropriate action. That's understandable.

The truth is, any doctor or surgeon learning anything new also has fear in the beginning. But once you get good at it, that fear is replaced by knowledge, skills and experience. Not to oversimplify, but it's almost like eating breakfast, lunch or dinner. You simply know how to do it. It's part of you. If I have to run to the hospital for an emergency procedure, there's no fear involved. It's that familiar to me.

So yes, any surgery presents some risk, but the patient should be fine. On the plus side, they'll be healthier as a result, and often feel better than they have in years!

Next I want to address some particular areas of heart health. A few were touched on early in this book. Others are subjects that you might never have considered, but I expect to be of great interest.

CHAPTER 33

WOMEN AND HEART DISEASE

Equality for All

Now that you have a better understanding of heart health, I want to explore the subject of women and heart disease in more detail.

As was briefly introduced in this book's fourth chapter, there is emerging awareness and concern today, as more women now die from coronary disease in this country each year than do men. If you really start to examine the numbers, you also discover that more women die of heart attacks than men within the same age groups. In fact, when women show up with their first heart attack, 52 percent of them die from sudden cardiac death. Men, 42 percent. This is true even if women don't have significant blockages in their vessels.

Some of the explanation behind this is women generally have more disease process than men. That is, the disease has actually progressed further without their necessarily being aware of it. This is partly because women don't seek out cardiology doctors as much as men do. They don't believe they're at as high a risk. Plus, when many doctors see female patients, *even they* don't treat them as aggressively as they do men. They underutilize the American Heart Association guidelines for treating women, which at the moment are identical for both sexes.

It is also possible for there to be small "silent" heart attacks prior to what's recognized as the "first attack" and a person not know it. These types of attacks go undetected more frequently in women, as most doctors still aren't anticipating heart disease like they do with men.

Additionally, there are circumstances linked to heart problems that are unique to women. A recent study showed that women who've experienced a stillbirth or repeated miscarriages have a greater chance of having heart attacks later in their lives. It was found that the risk of a heart attack for someone who's had at least one stillbirth was 3.5 times higher than for women who'd had none. Those who have experienced more than three spontaneous miscarriages had a fivefold increase in their likelihood of having a heart attack. (An induced abortion seemed to have no effect on the later likelihood of a heart attack.)

Furthermore, like men, women are not immune to stress impacting their heart health. A recent 10-year Harvard study found that women with high-stress jobs had a 40 percent higher risk of having some kind of heart disease, along with an 88 percent higher likelihood of experiencing a heart attack.

As suggested earlier, women's predisposition toward heart disease is not only a new perception for many doctors, it also contradicts the expectations of most women, who are generally more concerned about cancer than heart disease. This is despite statistics that show for women, one out of every 2.6 deaths in the U.S. is due to heart disease, while one out of every 4.6 females that dies is because of cancer.

Hormone Replacement Doesn't Work

We've long known that overall, men die earlier than women. Men have a lower life expectancy. One explanation behind this is has been that women's hormones, such as their higher levels of estrogen, protect them longer than men from various ailments.

But once women hit menopause, they basically catch up in terms of cardiology. The estrogen that had protected them diminishes. So doctors would administer hormone replacement therapy to compensate.

Then studies in 2002 found that the replacement therapy we'd been giving women – turns out not to protect them as once thought. It may actually *increase* a woman's chances of heart disease. Plus, it was deduced that hormone therapy may cause *other* serious problems, such as increased risk of breast cancer. Therefore, most of these therapies are no longer administered. This has been a great disappointment to many women, who depended on hormone replacement to compensate for many of the undesired changes that occurred during menopause.

So why don't hormones work?

Our bodies are normally in complete harmony. Perfectly put together. So if we find a person to be low in something, naturally we might conclude, "All right then, let's simply give it to them. That should solve it."

But it doesn't always work that simply.

The body is very complex, its many parts interconnected. We can't just assume, "This is at a low level so let's supplement it back up." Sometimes you can, but generally it's more complicated. Anything added can affect beyond the intended focus. That's partly why there are usually some side effects to most medications. We always have to decide if the benefits of the medication outweigh any risks posed by its side effects.

Another reason why research always continues.

Women have Different Symptoms

Another aspect of the misperception that women are less prone to heart disease than men are the differences in how symptoms show up in women and men. As said previously, symptoms can be invaluable clues to some condition in the body needing to be addressed. But women do not have the classic tell-tale symptoms of blockages that men have. An example is men with coronary disease typically experience angina when walking – the "classic" chest pressure and squeezing, radiating to the left side of the body and down their arm. But instead, women get what we call "angina equivalent." That can be pain in the upper back, fatigue, shortness of breath, or perfused sweating. It's not as dramatic or clear. And not as well-known.

In addition, if you look at women's heart arteries, you don't see as many high-grade blockages as in men's. Women don't tend to have arteries that are blocked in one area. If they have coronary disease, they tend to have diffused coronary artery disease. This means their artery isn't blocked in one specific area or another, but the whole vessel is diffusedly blocked. This is actually much harder to treat, as opposed to having one confined problem area where you can put in a stent and you're done.

Additional Dissimilarities

Aside from the already described disparities between women and men in connection to heart disease, women are also distinctly different in terms of:

- Microvascular Dysfunction
- Plaque Erosion
- Abnormal Coronary Reactivity
- Higher Cholesterol
- Calcium Scores
- CIMT Results
- Framingham Risk Assessment Results
- Response to Emotional Distress
- Likelihood of Obesity
- Vitamin D Deficiency

Let's take a look at these areas in more detail.

Microvascular Dysfunction

When comparing effects of heart disease on men and women, we have to factor in that women probably have more microvascular dysfunction (sometimes called microvessel disease). It's one reason that most women don't exhibit the same warning signs as men – their symptoms and pain are microvascular.

What does this mean?

We all have several large arteries that go around the heart. That's what we look at when performing angiograms. But as we go deeper into the body tissues, the blood pathways get smaller and smaller. Heart disease may not necessarily involve a big blockage in a big artery. It can be blockages down in this microvascular system (micro means very small). One might get good blood flow in the main artery, but not into the tissue. These microvessels typically control blood supply to the heart tissue during times of high demand, such as exercise or stress. Blockages in these can cause ischemia (decreased oxygen and nutrients to tissue). If lasting long enough while demand is high, a heart attack can result.

This appears to be more of an issue for women than men. One explanation is that the variances in hormone levels throughout a woman's life (changing during pregnancy to peripartum to menopause), all can raise the risk of more microvascular disease.

So women may not have big blockages in main arteries on top of the heart as much as they have tiny ones inside muscles and organs. These microvascular blockages actually create more symptoms, but doctors can't figure out *why* the patient is having them. Treadmill stress tests and angiograms don't typically pick up problems in microvessels. They'll indicate the person is fine, when in truth, they are not. As a result, many women coming in with this problem will be told they're not candidates for treatment. But if your doctor isn't concerned about these symptoms that you bring in, you might bring this possible explanation to their attention. They may not be as up-to-date on these recent discoveries.

Doctors current on the latest research – realizing a patient has symptoms, but an angiogram shows no blockages – will understand there's a possibility of microvascular disease. Some treatments that may help are statin drugs, which help to control cholesterol, and in turn improve function in the inner linings of the arteries. ACE inhibitors can also help improve function of the arteries' inner linings, as well as microcirculation.

There are still many questions about this condition, though it helps explain why women generally have worse outcomes and more deaths from cardiovascular disease.

Plaque Erosion

As described elsewhere, fat in the artery is called plaque. It adheres to an artery wall and builds up. Now, the blood moving through arteries normally has substances within it to keep everything thin and flowing, assuming there is not *too much* fat. In addition, the inside lining of the arteries work to keep everything flowing smoothly. But cholesterol can get under the smooth part of the artery and form plaque. This plaque can then become unstable and either erode or rupture into the artery. It's like having a foreign object inside your vessel. The body feels it must protect itself and clot over the object. But when a clot generates over it – and this happens fast – this can cause a heart attack. And there may be very little warning.

Two different types of plaque can cause thrombosis (blood clots). Because of estrogen, women under 50 tend to have plaque that is less dense without hardening on top, which is apt to *erode*. Women over 50 (and most men) tend to have a denser plaque with hardening on top that leads to *rupture*.

That's why with heart attack patients, we immediately give numerous blood thinners to eliminate any blood clotting, and go into the artery to place a stent at the blockage to keep the vessel open.

Another clot-forming tendency with women, aside from plaque erosion, is they may develop smaller clots on the surface of a large vessel, which then separate and flow through the blood to block smaller vessels further down.

Coronary Reactivity

Women can also have what we call abnormal coronary reactivity. It means their vessels react differently than normal under stress. For example, under general stress, they are more prone to have spasms of the arteries. They may not necessarily have a clot or blockage, but because of stress-related issues, they're more prone to these arterial spasms that cause less blood flow to the heart and possibly chest pains. If severe enough and continuing long enough, these spasms can even cause a heart attack.

The cardiovascular profiler test accesses the reactivity of the artery, how well it dilates (expands) and contracts. That by itself can reveal problems with the inner linings of the arteries.

Higher Cholesterol

Women also tend to have higher cholesterol than men. Within that cholesterol, they also tend to have lower HDL (the good cholesterol). Additionally, high triglycerides tend to more negatively affect women in terms of causing blockages and heart attacks.

Calcium Score

Women are frequently concerned about calcium levels in their bones as they age. But I refer to another kind of calcium here that has nothing to do with the calcium in your bones, what you take in supplements, or in the dairy you consume.

When you get plaque inside your arteries, it can go under the vessel wall, build up, and become *calcified*. This is of concern. In fact, when we do a CAT scan of someone, we can predict the risk of heart disease from the amount of calcium we find in the heart.

When you develop plaque inside the arteries, it can have different types of "remodeling." Normally it can remodel so it goes *outward* from the artery. You can have blockages, but it's not really blocking inside the artery. You can pick that up with the calcium score. But eventually, it becomes negative remodeling and goes inside the artery, which creates block-ages. Now you have an obstruction in the artery.

Calcium scores vary from zero into the 1000s. Different lev-els predict the likelihood of developing heart disease over the next 10 years. It's a good screening test, especially for patients who are borderline risks (like having a positive family history or being diabetic).

It is significant for women if they're at high risk from the calcium score, as chances for them developing heart disease or heart attacks are consequently 10 percent more than for men.

CIMT

Another difference in women and men is their CIMT results. Discussed in Chapter 29, CIMT measures the thickening of the inside lining of the neck's carotid artery that goes to the brain. Typically, if that result is normal, we measure the risk at only one percent. But if it turns out higher than what should be for someone of a certain age, the risk of having a blockage and a heart attack in the next 10 years will be much higher than if it was normal. That is generally true equally for men or women.

However, as the *thickness increases*, the risks are much higher in women than men.

Limits of the Framingham Risk Assessment

There is another reason why women may not be diagnosed as early with heart issues as men.

An evaluation referred to as the Framingham Risk Assess-ment is commonly used to compare variables such as age, sex, total cholesterol, HDL cholesterol, blood pressure and whether you smoke. It's designed to determine if you are at low or high risk for developing heart disease or attacks in the future.

But it undercuts some of the biomarkers particular to women. This is especially significant, since if the score comes out relatively low, some doctors may not perform further screening tests. In truth, it's not a good protocol to follow for any patient, as more recent studies show that by only using the Framingham Risk Assessment, 84 percent of patients marked as being low risk turned out to have significant blockages.

A newer assessment, called Reynolds Risk Score, would be a better choice. This assessment is more male/female specific, and considers the following variables:

- age
- gender
- systolic blood pressure
- CRP
- Total Cholesterol
- HDL
- Hemoglobin A1C (a marker for diabetes)
- smoking
- family history

Utilizing this formula, we're better able to detect early heart disease in women.

Broken Heart

By this, I don't literally mean the heart is "broken." That's certainly not a scientific medical term. But there is something referred to as "broken heart syndrome." As you might imagine, it refers to an emotional sorrow.

It is most often used to describe the condition of an elderly woman with recent emotional distress who has a heart attack. We do an ultrasound and see that half of the heart isn't working. But an angiogram shows no blockage, and the blood enzyme that we look at to judge how much damage was done to the heart doesn't register very highly. Then in a few months, the heart is better again.

Everything looks like a heart attack, but there are absolutely no blockages. Yet it's actually a heart attack. What probably occurred was that the heart wasn't getting enough oxygen, but then in a few moments the heart goes back to normal. The muscle is acutely damaged, though not bad enough to last an extensive time.

So is there an emotional connection? Does "sadness in the heart" somehow affect it physically? Science is still searching for those answers.

Weighty Subject

Another factor more emphasized in women is weight. The obesity epidemic in this country appears to be striking women more than men. So much so, that women fashion retailers are beginning to cater to overweight and obese clientele as part of mainstream clothing lines, as two-thirds of the female population is thought to fall into these categories. As previously addressed, obesity is a risk factor for developing heart disease (as well as diabetes).

Vitamin D Deficiency

It is commonly agreed there is a general deficiency of vitamin D in women today. Some feel it's due to inadequate diets. Others point out that many women no longer get sufficient sunlight exposure (which causes vitamin D to synthesize in the skin) – perhaps another consequence of our modern tendency to lead sedentary, *indoor* lives.

We know that vitamin D plays a significant role in healthy bones. Additional research indicates its deficiency may increase risks of certain cancers in women, as well as negatively affect the immune system and inflammatory illnesses.

A recent study, however, also points to vitamin D deficiency in younger women possibly elevating risks of high blood pressure in mid-life. The premenopausal women in the study with this vitamin deficiency were *three times* more likely to have systolic hypertension 15 years later, when contrasted to others with normal vitamin D levels. (Another recent study also showed that vitamin D deficiencies double the chance of fatal strokes in both women and men in white populations. However, there was no such effect on African Americans).

While the causes behind much of all this are not yet fully understood, it can be concluded for the moment that women would be wise to get more vitamin D-producing sunshine, increase the amount of vitamin D-rich foods in their diets, or take supplements, consulting with their doctor as to appropriate amounts.

The Good News: Keep Good Thoughts

The myth that women are somehow more immune to coronary disease than men is clearly fading. Women need to be just as conscientious toward their health habits as do men, and similarly consult with a cardiologist when necessary. Their warning signs can be more diverse than the classic indicators, which means that in some cases, women may proactively need to "educate" their own doctors to current information as presented in this book.

But your health may be more within your control than even stated so far. A recent study curiously showed that women who were optimistic (believing in favorable outcomes) had lower probability of developing heart disease and dying than pessimistic women.

Studying post-menopausal women, researchers found the optimistic were nine percent less likely to develop heart disease than the pessimistic, with a 14 percent lower likelihood of dying. The differences were even more pronounced among African American women.

So far, researchers aren't clear if changing one's attitude will alter the risk of heart disease (it's something they simply haven't studied yet). Future research will tell us if negative attitudes affect men in the same way. But in the meantime, I suggest it is good advice for everyone to focus on nurturing a more positive attitude. It can only help to improve your health, and will undoubtedly generate a happier life – for yourself and those around you.

Fascinating New Theory

Speaking of creating a better existence for yourself and others around you…

New scientific study is pointing toward a woman's emotional and physical health not only influencing her own heart health – but also that of others.

Her children.

Surprising to many, current research is indicating that the quality of nutrition a fetus receives while in the womb – along with the pollutants, drugs and even infections that the mother is exposed to, as well as the mother's general and even emotional health – may affect her child's future health even when they are an adult! Some scientists even conjecture that perhaps many of today's illnesses – cardiovascular disease, hypertension, diabetes, cancer, allergies, obesity, and even mental and emotional problems – may have origins in the womb.

Specific to heart disease, there does appear to be a link between small birth size – which often points to poor prenatal nutrition – and heart disease as an adult in middle age. (This doesn't necessarily include premature babies, but rather those whose birth weight is significantly less than normal for their period of gestation.)

This is really interesting, because scientists have long believed heart disease was principally sourced from our genetics or poor health behaviors. But now there's a theory that when there is deficient prenatal nutrition, the fetus may shift more of the nutrients it does receive to the brain, thereby diminishing what goes to other parts of its body. This may bring about a weaker heart and vascular system in later years.

There are even theories being researched about subsequent long-term health effects on children of women who experience extreme stress or depression while pregnant. All of this certainly makes us want to pay more attention to the state of a mother's well-being and health habits during pregnancy.

If it is true that a mother can influence the future health of her unborn child *in a very positive manner,* her acting on that knowledge can be a great boon to her offspring for years to come! For example, scientists are exploring if it's possible that consuming broccoli or other cruciferous vegetables while pregnant, can give the child a better chance of warding off future cancers.

All this is certainly more motivation to adopt a healthy lifestyle while pregnant...which in turn might facilitate the mother to adopt a lifelong healthier lifestyle for herself!

At the moment, research continues. We will see what the future brings.

CHAPTER 34

THE ATHLETIC HEART
Sudden Cardiac Death in Athletes

Two years ago, I gave a major presentation in Stockton, California. I invited presidents and athletic trainers of high schools and colleges, managers and trainers of professional basketball and football teams, as well as Olympic competitors and football players. The event was also supported by the California Chapter of the American College of Cardiology. This was done to raise their awareness of sudden cardiac death in athletes, the subject that I introduced briefly in this book's fourth chapter.

What Happens During Sudden Cardiac Death?

These athletes die of arrhythmias. Actually, pretty much everyone dying from a heart problem does so from an arrhythmia.

Let me recap how the heart works, as explained earlier in Chapter 11. A correctly functioning heart has electrical activity going from the top of the heart to the bottom, making the heart squeeze and pump correctly. An arrhythmia is when the entire electrical portion of the heart is firing all at once. The muscle cannot function. The pumping fails. You pass out since you're not getting enough oxygen to the brain, and in time you die.

The most obvious sign of an arrhythmia is blacking out due to lack of blood pressure.

CPR doesn't really revive you. That *can* happen, but CPR really just keeps your heart pumping blood through your body by pressing down on the chest. This keeps you alive until paramedics or someone arrives to perform more intensive intervention (like with a defibrillator) to restore heart function. In fact, you should be aware that CPR isn't even always successful. It really needs to be performed *perfectly* to keep a patient alive. That's why staying practiced and updated on its ever-improving protocols is so vital. If you ever have the opportunity to learn or review your CPR skills – take it.

Fortunately, young athletes are generally very healthy. As soon as they're down, if you shock them with a defibrillator, their heart rhythm can restore. They come back very fast and are just like they were before. It's pretty astonishing.

Prevention as Solution

The bottom line that I gave at the presentation in our state capital was this: if we have a policy in place in which a competent physician evaluates all athletes before they start rigorous exercise activity, we can prevent many young athletes from abruptly collapsing and dying.

Others have already begun doing this. In Northeastern Italy, a simple EKG test has been added to the examination of all athletes. An EKG is a simple exam costing only around $30. They were especially motivated to try this, as there happened to be a fairly prevalent genetic condition in this region called ARVD. With this simple testing, they were able to cut down the risk of sudden cardiac death in their athletes by 85 percent!

I suggested we adopt using such a test in the United States as well. While there are more expensive tests one can do (like an echocardiogram), an EKG should be able to detect over 95 percent of those with the underlying conditions that could lead to sudden cardiac death.

I would also encourage athletes to be aware of the possible warning signs of sudden cardiac death (SCD), which include chest pain, palpations, feelings of passing out, and shortness of breath outside of the norm one would expect with exercise. If experiencing these symptoms, the person should be evaluated by a cardiologist knowledgeable about SCD in athletes.

The Solution on the Field

While prevention is key (as it is with all cardiology), something can also be done if an arrhythmia causes an athlete's collapse.

Aside from presenting information to athletic program professionals at conferences and elsewhere, I proactively chose to take another step to improve safety for school athletes. As discussed earlier, a terrific device called a defibrillator sends a therapeutic dose of electrical current into a person's body to normalize heart function in various life-threatening situations. It's what you've seen on TV and in movies, where paddles are placed on the patient's chest in a hospital or by paramedics, and the heart is "shocked" back into beating correctly.

In real life, if someone collapses and you get to them within five minutes and shock them out of arrhythmia, they will likely survive. But if it takes longer than five minutes to shock them in this manner, the likelihood of survival is almost zero. That's why *these devices need to be at athletic fields everywhere*. The time it takes for someone to phone for help, for paramedics to arrive and get to the student, break out the equipment and use it – will most likely exceed those precious five minutes.

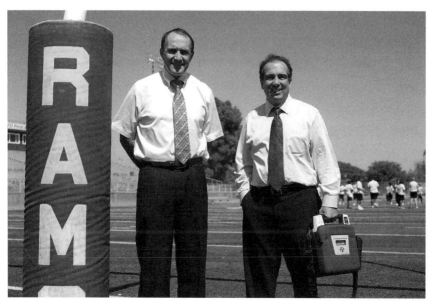

Holding portable defibrillator with Principal Morelli of Stockton's St. Mary's High School. Mr. Morelli is also an NFL referee

Portable Automatic Defibrillators

Fortunately, there are also portable "automatic" defibrillators. Even a person with little training can use one. You simply attach the leads to the chest, press the button, and it performs its own diagnosis and shock. So if someone collapses, you grab it and use it right away before paramedics even get there. If a portable automatic defibrillator is applied within the first minute, the survival rate is 90 percent. But if no such defibrillator is present, then survival drops to five percent, even with CPR. These defibrillators cost about $2000 each, but if one of these can save someone's life, they're worth *many* times that.

I felt it imperative that high schools possess these life-saving tools. I partnered with Dameron Hospital (CEO Chris Arismendi, MD), St. Jude Medical and Cardiac Science (a company that manufactures these high-end defibrillators) to put a program in place that would help provide automatic defibrillators to local high schools.

In addition, the proceeds from this book will go to help purchase portable automatic defibrillators for high schools as well.

Most recently, The Sacramento Kings basketball organization realized the importance of this program, and has been working with me to create a PSA (public service announcement) to raise awareness of sudden cardiac death in athletes. In fact, once the owners, Gavin and Joe Maloof, originally became aware of this project, they immediately got personally involved. Geoff Petrie, the General Manager, similarly offered to support the cause without hesitation. In addition, their media team has shown a genuine caring attitude in their assistance with this PSA. From this experience, I can truly say that we are fortunate to have such an organization in our community.

Athletics Offers Terrific Benefits

Though writing about a potential risk to athletes, I don't mean to scare anyone away from athletics. I'm actually a big proponent of sports, and believe they have immense value for young people.

Personally, I've always loved sports and have played many for fun. Competitively, I did wrestling, as well as track and field in high school. But my number one sport was soccer. I've played since I was five years old, and later in high school and college. I even played semi-pro in Sacramento, California, and also gave soccer camps. Most of those with whom I played have since gone on to play professionally somewhere in Europe (there were no professional teams here at that time).

Though I went into medicine instead, I find athletics has benefits far beyond the exercise and fitness. It has the positive effect of socialization, competitiveness and teamwork. Plus the sense of achieving a goal. I highly recommend every student-athlete be involved in some sport. Not necessarily to become a pro and earn money, but to develop these values that will help in their future and daily work lives.

Being competitive, while also being a gentleman or gentlewoman as an athlete, is an example of what I learned as a student-athlete that helped me be successful in life. Learning to be a team player assisted me in medical school, and helps me with my partners in my medical practice now. I trace it back to an important moment when a coach explained to me that even when you're in position to score, if your teammate is in better position, you pass it to him. You look better, he looks better, the whole team looks better. Today in the same way, if I'm in a position professionally to help my colleagues, I do it because then the whole group benefits.

I relate all this because even while there are risks in everything, there are distinct benefits as well. I wouldn't want some parent or student to shy away from participating in athletics because of anything I've presented here.

I simply feel it is my responsibility to relay health information like what I've described in this chapter, even if it makes some people uncomfortable. Perhaps that discomfort will motivate others to champion their own quest to enhance protections for our young athletes.

Knowledge is Powerful

On a larger note, I want the reader to receive the information offered throughout this book as something to benefit their well-being, not as cause for worry. While there are always conditions that can go wrong, the body is an amazing creation (have I said "amazing" *enough*?). It manages itself in remarkable ways.

Readers must simply be informed about their own body and how it functions, not just for their own sake, but for the sake of others too. If a person who's read this book sees someone experiencing a medical "event" as I've described, everyone else might stand around not knowing what happened (possibly thinking the fallen individual only had the wind knocked out of him). But my reader may jump into action. Start CPR while yelling for someone to call 911, or summon the proper equipment to resuscitate someone. Perhaps a person's life will be saved – simply because someone took the time to read these pages.

CHAPTER 35

WINTER RISKS

Tis the Season to be Jolly – and Careful

In some ways, people are more mindful of their general health during cold weather seasons. They may get flu shots. They make sure their hair is dry after washing before venturing outside. They buy winter coats.

What they don't realize is they also need to "bundle up" against heart attacks. Why? There are more heart attacks during winter than any other season. Comprehending why will also help you understand more about your body.

Your body has an intriguing response mechanism to deal with cold. The goal is to keep the core of your body at 98.6 degrees. One of the ways your body does this is by constricting blood vessels to limit the loss of body heat. This does help, but it also raises blood pressure and lowers the amount of blood flowing to your heart and other organs. If you are being active at the same time, this can put a significant demand on your heart. If you already have heart disease, it may be too much and cause a heart attack. That's why you hear warnings about the high risk of coronary events while shoveling snow.

So how might you protect yourself? For shoveling snow, you can hire others (hopefully those at less risk) to do it for you. Yes, there's cost involved. But certainly minor compared to chancing a heart attack. If you do go outside, make doubly sure you are warmly clothed, so your blood vessels have less tendency to contract in order to preserve heat. Cover your head, hands – all that you can. If you are shoveling, don't try to do too much at one time; take breaks frequently. Remember – snow is *heavy*. Not so much when hurling a snowball, but much more when shoveling. Also, be sure to stretch and warm up your body before going out, so your activity puts less strain on you.

When shoveling, be alert. Symptoms of a heart attack can seem similar to those for a pulled muscle, including squeezing or other pains in your chest area, or pain in your arms, back or neck. They can also include shortness of breath, sweating or nausea. Pay extra attention to any warning signs *after* shoveling too. If you feel chest pains, always take an aspirin immediately as this can dramatically decrease chances of dying from a heart attack. Any size aspirin will do, though if there is an acute sign of heart attack, again it is best to *chew* 325 mg of aspirin (a full strength aspirin).

CHAPTER 36

ON THE SUBJECT OF SEX...
Health Concerns and Erectile Dysfunction

People with coronary conditions naturally wonder if sex can put a strain on their heart.

It is possible. The general guideline is that walking up two flights of stairs equates to the strain on your heart while having a sexual encounter. In our practice, if the patient can make that climb without any significant shortness of breath or chest pain, we consider the likelihood of having difficulties from sex to be low. Not zero, but low.

So the healthier your heart, not only is the sex safer (we all want safe sex!), but also more enjoyable as you have increased stamina.

It should be pointed out that this concern doesn't only apply to older persons. I had one man in his thirties come in who was getting chest pains from having sex with his girlfriend. With this information and a full exam, I was able to find that he had a very high-grade blockage in his heart.

The pain he felt was an alert. A very *valuable* warning signal. I put a stent in his artery and afterwards he was fine. Suffice it to say, he was very grateful (I heard his girlfriend was as well).

Erectile Dysfunction

Hopefully by now it is apparent that issues with heart health can create other, seemingly non-related health issues. But a problem you still might not expect to be connected is erectile dysfunction. While this exclusively affects men, it in turn has consequences for women as well.

Also called impotence, erectile dysfunction refers to an inability to sufficiently maintain an erection to have sex. Occasional impotence isn't necessarily something to worry about, but a recurring problem can be another matter. It can negatively affect your sex life, your relationship, and even your self-esteem.

It may also be a sign of underlying medical problems.

While stress, tiredness, depression or relationship issues can also be the reason, there are a number of possible physical causes for impotence. Men with sexual problems of this nature are often smokers, people with high cholesterol or diabetes. Why? All of these affect the inner lining of the arteries. This can cause erectile dysfunction. It is the blood flowing through the arteries that feed the male organ. If you have blockages there, it may be obvious, as that can interfere with its function. But it doesn't take an actual blockage to affect the quality of your sex. High blood pressure can also impact the area. The sheer force of the pressure of the blood going to the vessels can damage the function of an artery. And if the artery isn't functioning well, then the organ will run into problems.

Many men have never suspected there's any correlation. In fact, many believe erectile dysfunction is simply something that often happens as they get older. But in truth, one of the main reasons this dysfunction occurs is that as men get older, their cholesterol levels have risen, and plaque has built up in the arteries. There are other factors as well. Testosterone and other hormones play a role. But the dysfunction for many relates directly to the condition of their vessels.

You'd be surprised how often I have patients come in who have this problem. But men being men, they don't say anything. They don't know to ask or are simply too embarrassed. Usually it's *the wife* who speaks up and asks, "Is there anything we can do?"

Fortunately…Yes

If you treat your underlying health issues by being active, eating right, not smoking and keeping your cholesterol down (and your sugar intake down if you have diabetes), you're more likely to have better function. Sure, it will take some effort. But the results are undeniably satisfying.

L-Arginine

If improving your health behaviors doesn't solve the problem, there are medications that doctors can prescribe. There is also an over-the-counter supplement that can assist. Called L-Arginine, it is an amino acid that has been shown in studies to improve function of the inner linings of arteries by helping the nitric oxide pathway. Not only can it potentially lower blood pressure, it has also been known to help correct erectile dysfunction. It should be noted that L-Arginine can interact with some other heart medications, including high blood pressure medicines known as ACE inhibitors, as well as nitroglycerin. So check with your doctor.

VIAGRA

Viagra is a medication commonly prescribed for erectile dysfunction (impotence) in men. While the best known, Viagra isn't the only one in this class of drugs. There is also Levitra and Cialis, both of which function similarly. All have been "miracle" drugs for many with this ailment. However, they also pose some very real concerns for those with heart conditions.

These types of drugs (phosphodiesterase inhibitors) work by inhibiting a particular enzyme in blood, thereby causing dilation of the vessel. When you have dilation of the vessel, the penis engorges with blood. That is how an erection forms.

Drug Interaction: Passing out and Heart attacks

There is a problem with using Viagra while taking nitrates. Nitrates are used by people who have chest pains. They're placed under the tongue to relieve the pain. But nitrates also cause vasal dilation, and the Viagra intensifies their effect. When you have too much vasal dilation, your blood pressure drops, you don't get enough blood flow to the brain and you can pass out.

A different problem can occur as well. If you vasodilate the arteries too much, they open up and the heart muscle itself doesn't get enough blood. If you already have some kind of blockage there, and suddenly have a supply/demand mismatch (more demand than supply), not enough blood flows to the heart muscle due to the lowered supply. It can precipitate a heart attack. In general, you should not take Viagra within 24 hours of any nitrates.

Other than Drug Interference...is Viagra Safe?

A patient might ask, "Should I have a workup done on my heart before I take any of these drugs?"

In general, there are two types of patient population: those with known heart disease and those without known disease. Of course, people without any *known* heart disease still might wonder if they can take the drug. To answer that, they can do a simple self test. If you can go up one flight of stairs without significant chest pain or shortness of breath, you should be fine taking this drug.

On the other hand, if you do have heart disease, your cardiologist should make a recommendation whether you can take the drug, based on the status of your condition. For instance, if you have single vessel disease, meaning you have one blockage that's been opened up by stenting, then you should be able to use Viagra. But if someone has multiple vessel blockages, or diffused disease in arteries that have not been corrected, then probably best not to use this drug. Once full blood flow has been restored to the heart and the patient has no more symptoms of chest pain or significant shortness of breath, then it should be safe.

Even given the above information, I would always have a patient ask their doctor before using this drug, rather than simply rely on the patient's recollection or understanding about the specifics of their condition. Plus, no two patients are exactly the same. What I'm giving are just guidelines. So final advice: consult your physician.

CHAPTER 37

MEDICATIONS

The Leading Edge

Heart medications are indispensible in helping patients with various conditions that might otherwise be life-threatening. They are frequently used in place of much more invasive and risky surgery. An interventional cardiologist myself, I always prefer to use a medication whenever possible in place of surgical procedures.

I also feel very fortunate to be on the forefront of research for treatment with medications. I speak for many of the companies manufacturing these drugs, often at seminars teaching other cardiologists. So I'm always being updated on the latest discoveries – not only about new drugs, but also about drugs already in use. While I am paid for giving these presentations, I don't simply do it for the money. I have to believe in the medication. I've turned down offers when I didn't feel comfortable about the benefits of a particular drug.

Practically every two weeks, I'm traveling someplace to meet directly with research personnel at the companies that make these drugs. They update me on their latest information and studies, as well as ask my thoughts about products, tapping into my experience using the drugs that already exist.

The biggest benefit to all of this is that I learn the latest about medications. Then I use my own judgment and clinical experience to utilize or not utilize drugs to deliver the best quality care to patients.

Variety

Fortunately, there are wide selections of drugs that cardiologists can use to help people who have heart problems – or help to avoid them. The reason for this diversity is the existence of different classes of drugs for different issues. These include:

- hypertension drugs
- cholesterol medications
- anti-angina drugs
- anti-arrhythmic drugs
- blood thinning drugs

There are others as well. It should give people with heart conditions some comfort to know that as doctors determine the cause of their problem, they can choose the most effective drug to counter it.

Side Effects

As wonderful as many of these medications are, you should be aware that no drug is perfect. Though some are as close as can be to perfect.

As with almost all medications, there can be side effects, some more serious than others. As frequently cited in this book, the human body is amazingly complex and its many parts intertwined. You make an adjustment in one area of the body, there are chances it will shift something in another. That's the nature of medicine.

This isn't true only with medications. Even over the counter supplements can have unexpected side effects. Take vitamin E, for example. For some time, many have believed it was beneficial to heart health. There is some truth to this. A recent study confirmed that vitamin E can lower the risk of Ischemic strokes – a mild kind of stroke – by 10 percent. But the study *also* found that vitamin E *raises* the risk of a more severe kind of stroke (hemorrhagic) by 22 percent. This points to the perils of "self-treating." Given these results, the study's researchers cautioned against the random use of vitamin E.

It would be appropriate to point out that when heart medications are criticized because of their side effects – it's very often when they are given in fairly high doses. Yet there are ways to keep dosage levels lower. One of those is with combination therapy.

Combination Therapy

It's noteworthy that patients sometimes wonder why a doctor may prescribe more than one medication for a condition. It's really not that we're trying to sell them on more drugs. A combination of drugs is actually more effective. Many studies have backed this up, as hardly anyone's disease is controlled with one medication. Let me explain.

First, as has been said previously, the body is an intricate mechanism. There can be more than one cause behind a medical condition. But beyond even this, there's another compelling reason to use more than one drug.

In this country, there's a common attitude that "more is better." So some might expect that if a drug has some benefit to a patient, then increasing the dosage will increase the benefit. But often that is not the case. Studies have found that it doesn't matter if you're taking blood pressure or cholesterol medication; in general, the *most benefit* you get is with the *first lowest dose*. That is, increasing the dosage of the medication *doesn't* mean you get the same proportionate benefit. As example, with cholesterol drugs, every time you double the dosage, you only decrease cholesterol by six percent. You get the greatest benefit – generally over a 25 percent decrease – with the first low dosage.

Plus, anytime you increase the dosages of medications, *you increase the chance for side effects.* So it is generally better to use combinations of drugs, each at lower dosages to yield fewer side effects.

Choosing the Best Drug

As you will see in these chapters, there are numerous drugs available to choose from for most every ailment. So how do we select the right one? Essentially, there are three main traits to a drug's appropriateness:

- Is it efficacious? Meaning, does it produce the desired effect?
- Is it easy to use? Must it be taken once per day? Twice? More?
- Is it low or high in side effects (called the side effect profile)?

If you have a drug possessing the best of all these three traits, it is probably the best drug in its class.

CHAPTER 38

HYPERTENSION DRUGS
Depressurizing High Blood Pressure

When someone's blood pressure goes up, there's a variety of possible reasons. Fortunately, we have a variety of drugs to deal with every cause.

In fact, there are different *classes of drugs* just for hypertension. They each function in different parts of the body, with a different mechanism of action, in order to match and counteract whatever is raising the blood pressure.

My favorite hypertensive drugs are in the RAAS blockade category, which affect the neuro-hormonal cascade in our body that starts with our kidneys. To understand these drugs, it's helpful to understand what they are treating.

The RAAS System

RAAS refers to the renin-angiotensin-aldosterone – a hormone system based in the kidneys that helps control blood pressure and blood volume in your body. I addressed it briefly in this book's seventh chapter. How it actually works is sort of an education in the complexities of our bodies.

When the volume of your blood is low (as could happen if bleeding from an injury), the kidneys secrete renin. This renin in turn activates production of angiotensin, which causes constriction of your blood vessels. This "cascade" of responses ends up increasing the blood pressure, as it's supposed to. Not only that, the angiotensin also causes the adrenal cortex to release another hormone, aldosterone, which amplifies the reabsorption of water and sodium in the blood. In effect, this increases blood volume and pressure.

In other words…wow.

A fantastic system. However, if for some reason this renin-angiotensin-aldosterone system remains activated when it's not needed, as sometimes happens in hypertensive patients, your blood pressure rises too much. The various drugs in the RAAS system work to disrupt different portions of this RAAS cascade, in order to help reduce the blood pressure back down.

RAAS Blockade Drugs

I favor drugs in this class because studies have shown they not only reduce blood pressure, they also have *secondary positive effects* on the body, such as reducing heart attacks, strokes, and onset of diabetes. These wider positive effects are due to the drug improving the function of the inner lining of the arteries.

So what are the drugs within this RAAS group?

• Ace Inhibitors
• ARB Class
• Renin Inhibitor

Ace Inhibitors

Ace inhibitors have been available for many years and extensively studied. They have great beneficial effect not only for hypertension, but also for prevention and delay of diabetes causing damage to the kidneys. It also helps those with congestive heart failure to live longer and healthier.

My concern with these drugs is there's a chance they'll cause a dry hacking cough in up to 30 percent of patients. It's curious that in my practice, patients seldom bring up experiencing this side effect until I mention it. If they do confirm having it, then I switch to another drug and the cough goes away. So again, my advice for patients is always to be more proactive in knowing about this possible side effect, and letting their doctors know if they experience this cough.

ARB Drugs

The next in the RAAS group are the ARB class of drugs (angiotensin receptor blockers).

The first example of this drug came out around 1994. Called Cozaar, the benefit of this drug over the previous types is that it works one step further in the cascade. Side effects are lower with this drug than ace inhibitors too. Patients have less chance of having a dry cough. We can't say zero chance, but much lower. Also, some people experience swelling of the tongue and mouth from ACE inhibitors, which is less likely with this drug.

Very well-tolerated, the ARB drugs are similar to the ACE inhibitors in that they also can beneficially lower the progression of diabetic neurotrophy – the worsening of kidney function that leads to dialysis. Studies also show that ARB drugs enhance endothelial function (inner lining of the vessel), which means less chance of heart attacks and strokes.

It's important to note that all of these RAAS cascade drugs should be *avoided by women during pregnancy*, as the medication can affect the development of the embryo's kidneys. They should also be avoided by people with very advanced kidney disease, and should only be taken with the consult with a kidney doctor (nephrologist) and a cardiologist together.

Direct Renin Inhibitors (DRI Drugs)

Some new drugs have appeared in the last few years. A prominent example is Tekturna. Also called Aliskiren, it is a direct renin inhibitor that works right at the start of the whole RAAS cascade, blunting the overactivation right from the beginning.

There are additionally some hormonal benefits to this, but the extent of those benefits is still under research. Basically, it has given cardiologists an extra method of lowering blood pressure, which is valuable since in general, we cannot lower blood pressure with just one drug. Almost everybody needs two to four drugs to lower blood pressure.

Combinations

There are some combinations of hypertension medications I find especially effective. The best combinations are a RAAS class with a diuretic, or a RAAS class with a calcium channel blocker (I will describe both diuretics and calcium channel blockers in more detail in later sections).

A RAAS system drug – one of the ACE, ARB or DRIs – in addition to a low dose diuretic like HCTZ (Hydrochlorothiazide), offers greater effectiveness in lowering blood pressure than can be had by increasing dosages on either drug (and risking increased side effects). By the same token, these same RAAS blockade drug classes used with a calcium channel blocker like Norvasc is a very effective combination too.

In fact, some companies manufacture medications that are *already a combination of two drugs.* There is an ACE inhibitor and a calcium channel blocker combination drug called Lotrel (mixture of Benazepril and Norvasc). A drug called Azor is a blend of an ARB and a channel blocker (Benicar and Norvasc).

There's also a combination drug called Exforge (Diovan and Norvasc), as well as Twynsta (Micardis and Norvasc).

As illustration of ever-evolving and improving medications, there's another combination drug called Valturna that's entirely within the RAAS system that came out recently. It was the first drug to combine the ARB Class and the DRI together (Aliskiren and Valsartan). It yields even more of a blockade of the RAAS System, creating double digit reductions in blood pressure. It's a well-tolerated medication, as the potential side effects are very similar to those of ARB and DRI together.

Again, these combinations offer more potency in reducing blood pressure, are more user-friendly to the patient (who's thinking psychologically he's taking only one drug rather than two), and offer less side effects.

Calcium Channel Blockers

Calcium channel blockers work differently than the RAAS classification of drugs. They lower blood pressure by dilating (opening) the vessels. Relaxing the smooth muscle cells within the vessel walls, they cause the vessels to widen and thus lower the pressure. They are particularly effective for elderly patients with isolated systolic hypertension (referring to only the top number in blood pressure being elevated – normally 120/80).

First Generation

The first generation of calcium channel blockers includes Cardizem and Verapamil. They're very effective, but can have the side effect of edema (swelling) in the legs. With Verapamil, you may get constipation too. These drugs also cause the heart muscle to beat less strongly (not necessarily preferred, though this does reduce blood pressure), and therefore are sometimes used for people with chest pains as it lowers the demand on the heart. They are also given to those with arrhythmias, as it can also lower the heart rate. These drugs are mostly used for people who have emphysema, and cannot tolerate beta blockers (another type of drug that will be described) for their arrhythmias. We use them only in low doses. In high dosages, some people get fatigued because the heart is not working as robustly as it normally would.

Second Generation

The second generation of calcium channel blockers is called dihydropyridines. They do not have the negative effects of making the heart weaker or slowing its rate, but they maintain the desired effect of vasal dilation that opens up the arteries to lower blood pressure. The benefit of this is that it can be used safely in patients with many different types of diseases, such as heart failure, coronary disease and chest pains.

The only problem with these drugs is that they carry a high tendency for edema, especially at higher doses. However, when you use them at low dose in combination with a drug from the RAAS class, you get better reduction of blood pressure and fewer side effects. To illustrate, studies have shown that if you increase dosages from five milligrams of Norvasc to ten milligrams, the risk of edema is significant – approximately 30 percent. *But* if you use the drug at five milligrams with another drug from the RAAS class, the likelihood of edema goes down dramatically, and you get the same or even more blood pressure reduction than if you had raised the dihydropyridines to the higher dose.

Beta Blockers

Beta Blockers have been around for over 30 years. In fact, they were one of the first medications created to lower blood pressure. The prototype beta blocker was Propanol.

Yet it's not exactly known how it reduces blood pressure, except that we know it lowers the demand on the heart, thus allowing the heart to work less intensely. It also lowers the *"adrenergic drive"* that can bombard the heart and vessels. "Adrenergic" refers to the "fight or flight syndrome." That is where the person perceives physical danger, and the body releases hormones like norepinephrine to rev up your body (to either fight or flee). It makes you go-go-go! It *also* raises your blood pressure.

In a way, this mechanism responds similarly to much of the same stimuli as when the RAAS system over-activates if the body anticipates being injured. Chronic stress in our lives is interpreted by the body as a constant low-level threat, elevating our levels of norepinephrine. In some ways, you could suggest the necessity of beta blockers is in response to the constant stress levels in our modern times.

Blocking Reception

Interestingly, the beta blockers don't block the release of these hormones. Instead, they block the *receptors* these hormones would affect. By blocking the site where the hormone would be working, blood pressure doesn't rise. However, because the beta blockers make the heart beat less intensely, people can feel tired or sleepy, and even sometimes experience impotence.

Yet there is now a beta blocker that doesn't create those side effects. One of the latest and greatest (in my opinion) among the various beta blocker drugs is Bystolic, the newest dilating beta blocker. Unlike other beta blockers that only cause the heart to beat less intensely (and possibly cause people to feel tired, etc.), Bystolic at the same time dilates (opens up) the artery to take the workload off the heart as well. The two results cancel each other out in a way, so you don't have the side effects of fatigue, etc. That's why we don't have as many side effects with this drug as with older beta blockers. Bystolic also doesn't negatively affect insulin sensitivity or the lipid profiles (LDL, HDL and triglycerides) on people with diabetes, as can some older beta blockers.

Another vasal dilating beta blocker is called Coreg. It also has been shown to have no negative effects on cholesterol for people with diabetes. But it operates differently that Bystolic. Coreg uses the muscle within the artery to make it dilate, while Bystolic works at the endothelium (inner lining of blood vessels) though nitric oxide pathways. Bystolic's is a more physiologic way to dilate the artery – that is, it uses the natural way in which the artery itself functions to dilate on its own.

Overall, beta blockers are used in hypertension, and with people who've had heart attacks, heart failure, arrhythmias and atrial fibrillation. Each of the different beta blockers has different research results, so each one has different FDA approval for when it should be used, based on research thus far. For instance, Bystolic is fairly new and only approved for hypertension at this point. For Coreg, because it has been out longer (since around 2000), more studies have been completed with more FDA approvals granted. It has FDA approval for hypertension, as well as heart failure and for people after a heart attack. But I fully expect they'll find Bystolic to be effective for other heart conditions in the future.

Diuretics

Diuretics are another class of drugs used to lower blood pressure. They all work with the kidneys to reduce the amount of fluids (the water portion) in the arteries and veins, with the "unwanted" fluid taken out through the kidneys and bladder to be released as urine.

Less fluids circulating in the blood will mean less pressure. But you have to be careful not to overdo it. It has to be the right amount in order not to cause problems. It's now a fairly archaic way to lower blood pressure.

CHAPTER 39

CHOLESTEROL MEDICATIONS

Improving Your Blood

Aside from diet and exercise, cholesterol levels are largely controlled by medication. In the "old days," niacin supplements and bile acid sequestrants were the main classes of medications used to treat cholesterol. But everything changed once statin drugs were created in 1987.

Landmark studies in the early 1990s showed over and over that statins significantly lowered the risk of illness and death from heart disease and stroke, especially for people after they've had a heart attack.

While science can provide us remarkable and swift advancements in treatments, attitudes sometimes take a little longer to transform. I remember during my internal medicine residency (before I began my fellowship in cardiology), my professor would say, "Older patients in their 80s shouldn't be treated for high cholesterol, given their already advanced age." The belief then was that it took too long to effectively lower cholesterol levels to benefit people in this age bracket. Statin – the new "miracle drug" – wasn't for everybody.

It's amazing how that viewpoint has dramatically shifted. Today, we know that even in the short term, not only do statin drugs lower cholesterol, but they also stabilize the plaque. It actually makes the fat content within the artery more compact, rather than soft and more pliable where it can rupture and cause heart attacks and strokes.

Patients get immediate benefit from these drugs even beyond the longer term advantages of lowering cholesterol levels. Statins also lower the markers of heart disease, such as CRP (explained previously as a marker of the amount of vascular blockages in your body). This is the reason why studies have shown that *all diabetics,* regardless of their LDL cholesterol levels (even if within normal range), should be on statins. This is important.

Cholesterol Discoveries Along the Way

It is fascinating how cardiology has progressed over time. For instance, when doctors were first emphasizing the lowering of cholesterol, many believed that simply reducing levels 20 to 30 percent was the goal. Reducing further, they believed, didn't have significant benefit.

Then there was a big study, simply and appropriately entitled, "Prove It." The research was largely designed to see whether Pravachol or Lipitor was the more effective statin drug. But this study also revealed it was better to lower cholesterol levels *more* than the 20 to 30 percent as originally thought.

That's why today, we push patients to lower cholesterol further. In my own practice, I've found that patients who have previously had blockages, who then lower their LDL to 70, are much less likely to come back with more blockages. But those that don't adjust their lifestyle and diet, and don't take their medication, often return with blockages where I must go in surgically to put in stents.

Yet the benefit to lowering cholesterol isn't simply to avoid surgery. Patients can *feel better* due to decreased mental stress. They know they are much less likely to experience another heart attack or need a cardiologist to surgically repair their arteries. Time and again, I've witnessed people's faces suddenly brighten when their blood work reveals their levels have reduced.

Their quality of life *instantly* improved.

Which Statin for Which Patient?

By the way, the study I just cited ultimately showed Lipitor to more potent than Provachol. So does this mean everyone should be given Lipitor?

In a word, no.

Different drugs – and different potencies – are appropriate for different people. Pravachol would today be considered a mildly potent statin. Moderately potent would be Lipitor, Simvastatin and Zocor. High potency statin drugs are Crestor and Vytorin. Those last two are my "big guns," that we give to appropriate patients to more significantly lower their cholesterol levels.

The choice of drug and its potency largely relates to how much we need to lower someone's cholesterol level. Everyone has a goal regarding what level to which we should reduce their LDL, depending on their disease situation. As said earlier, for diabetics with at least one other risk factor (like high blood pressure or smoking), the recommendation is that their LDL should go down to 70. That number 70 is now actually the recommendation for all people with known vascular disease.

Statin Side Effects

There are patients that for one reason or another, cannot tolerate statins. Some people are very genetically prone to these side effects, while others are not. Side effects of statins can include muscle aches and pains, or muscle weakness.

Taking an over-the-counter supplement called Coenzyme Q10 (CoQ10), will sometimes diminish this muscle ache. It actually can help stop the muscles (including the heart muscle) from being weakened from statins. Basically it replenishes the ATP needed to transport energy within cells for metabolism that may get depleted by statin drugs. If a patient experiences aches and pains, or weakness in their muscles, they should consult their doctor about taking CoQ10.

Another possible side effect is that blood work might show a bump in liver enzymes – the result of statins modifying how the liver is functioning in order to lower cholesterol. That's why we must check liver function every three to six months when someone is on one of these drugs. But this side effect doesn't happen often. Only two to three percent of my patients have had elevated liver enzymes. Mild elevation isn't of serious concern under the guidelines. But since we can never know how something might affect an *individual patient*, to be on the safe side we usually try switching them to another drug that doesn't cause liver enzyme elevation.

I should point out that having treated thousands and thousands of patients using statins, I haven't had one end up with liver damage. This belief that statins will harm your liver has been exaggerated well out of proportion to reality, as long as your doctor periodically monitors your liver function. So make sure your doctor is having your liver function checked, and make sure *you go in* for the testing.

The statin drugs that don't work through the liver at all are bile acid sequestrants, like Welchol. As a result, they don't affect the liver nor require enzyme monitoring.

Welchol

A newer formulation of bile acid sequestrants, Welchol, came on the market in the early 2000s. It's pretty intriguing how Welchol lowers cholesterol in the bloodstream.

Cholesterol comes into your bloodstream in two different ways. One is through the food you eat. The other is from the liver, which actually manufactures cholesterol for various body needs.

As you eat, your body secretes bile to digest the food. Produced by the liver, bile is composed partially of cholesterol. When you take Welchol, it binds this bile acid, so it exits out the body through your digestion as opposed to being reabsorbed. So with Welchol, the liver then has to direct more of the cholesterol it produces to help make this bile acid. This way, we're indirectly reducing the amount of cholesterol the liver otherwise would make that goes into the bloodstream.

There is an issue with bile acid sequestrants if you already have high triglycerides, as it has some tendency to raise triglyceride levels. Also, if you have a problem with constipation, you wouldn't use Welchol, as that problem can be intensified. Other than this, Welchol is very safe. You take it within half an hour of your lunch or dinner, as that's when bile acid is released in the body.

However, Welchol only creates a 15 percent reduction in cholesterol. Sometimes I put people on both Welchol and a drug called Zetia, as you get about 15 percent cholesterol reductions with each. At that point, you've come close to the statins' ability for reducing cholesterol.

Zetia

The next class of drugs also came out during the early 2000s and is called Zetia. It's actually been getting some negative attention in the literature, as recent studies show that when comparing Zetia and niacin, niacin was slightly more potent in reversing any increased thickness of the carotid artery than Zetia. But we can still use Zetia, especially since it works very well in combination with statins to lower the LDL even further. It also doesn't have the side effects that can go along with niacin – the itching and flushing.

Plus, for patients who cannot tolerate statins, I often use Zetia as it lowers cholesterol levels 15 to 20 percent by itself. Instead of working in the liver like statins, Zetia works at the level of the small bowel, to help prevent absorption of the cholesterol from foods we eat.

But please note: while it does help limit cholesterol absorption, taking Zetia *doesn't* mean a patient can return to eating all the cholesterol-laden foods they may previously have been consuming. They still must improve their diet.

Fenofibrates

Fenofibrates are another class of drugs used to treat high cholesterol and high triglyceride levels. The prototype for the first ones is called Gemfibrozil. It lowers triglycerides and slightly raises HDL (good cholesterol). As always, we want to bring down the LDL (bad cholesterol) levels. But a study that came out during the early 2000s, showed you can significantly lower heart disease, heart attacks and strokes when you lower triglycerides and slightly raise HDL with these drugs.

The one fenofibrate approved by the FDA to be used safely along with statins is Trilipix. You still always have to guard for drug interaction between these two (increased muscle aches and pains), but because of the benefits, everyone uses them in combination. Your doctor just has to watch it even more closely.

The benefits are the LDL is lowered by the statin, and you lower triglycerides and raise HDL with the fenofibrate. Lowering triglycerides and raising HDL also affects the whole cholesterol cascade, and can thereby change the form of the LDL from type B (bad), to type A (much better).

Lovaza

As I wrote earlier, the last few years have seen a way to treat patients through what is essentially concentrated fish oil. Called Lovaza, it's basically polyunsaturated omega-3. Very heart healthy.

Lovaza is really for those with high triglycerides, and those with detailed LDL tests that show too much of the bad type B. Again, by lowering triglycerides, you promote more of the preferred type A LDL. Research also shows that Lovaza can raise HDL by nine percent.

Sometimes patients raise the question, "If Lovaza is really fish oil, then why don't we just use one of the fish oils sold over the counter?" The answer is that most of those fish oils are contaminated with mercury and are not highly purified. Lovaza is FDA approved with a five-step purification process. It is also much more *concentrated* than the fish oil available over-the-counter, and has been proven to lower triglycerides by 48 percent. That is *very* significant.

So for patients reluctant to take a drug, I say they now can take something that's natural, highly purified, with no side effects. It's one of those cases where science has improved upon what nature provides. One Lovaza pill equals six to thirteen (depending on the brand) of the over-the-counter versions of fish oil. So you take just two capsules of Lovaza, twice per day.

We continue to search for more uses for omega-3s like those in Lovaza. Some studies have shown high doses can lower risk of dying from sudden cardiac death. Other research shows omega-3s to have some anti-inflammatory benefits at high doses as well. As I discussed in Chapter 17, rheumatoid arthritis patients have significantly reduced symptoms by using high doses of Lovaza.

Niacin and Niaspan

Just as science was able to improve the effectiveness of omega-3 fish oil in Lovaza, there's a more potent and controlled formulation of the B-vitamin niacin, available in the drug Niaspan.

A fairly common vitamin, niacin has long been used to control cholesterol, primarily by increasing your HDL, as well as lowering LDL's bad component, LPa. In fact, niacin is the only "supplement" that lowers LPa in our system. To a mild degree, it can also reduce triglycerides. Additional studies have also shown it can stabilize and decrease the thickness of plaque inside vessels. Very multi-purpose in terms of cholesterol.

Over-the-counter niacin works somewhat in this regard, and there also exists a longer acting time-release niacin. But it's yet to be proven beneficial in this form, and has been shown to potentially cause liver problems.

The most effective of all is the prescription form, Niaspan, which is superior because it is more precisely regulated, such that we know the exact ingredients and amounts we're dealing with. It is more effective in controlling cholesterol, triglycerides, and reducing plaque thickness in blood vessels. Plus, remember when I described that LPa is much more potent than LDL in causing plaque to develop inside the artery? Niaspan is the only drug out there to lower LPa. Exercise, diet – nothing else reduces it. So if you have high LPa, this is your only solution.

The only problem with this drug is that significant numbers of people experience flushing, and possibly itching – both a common side effect of niacin as well. What happens during flushing is that your more superficial vessels – those near the skin – dilate and your skin turns red. There's no health risk, but it can be unpleasant. The other point to convey is that Niaspan also works through the liver, so your doctor should monitor liver function through periodic blood work.

We've found that the higher the dose of Niaspan, the better the results. But that also increases likelihood of side effects. At 500 milligrams, side effects of flushing and itching are very low. But as you move up to 1000 or 2000 milligrams, side effects become more pronounced. We advise patients to reduce the risk of flushing by taking their aspirin (in this case, higher 325 mg aspirin is preferred) a half hour after taking their Niaspan. We even go one step further, by suggesting a patient take their Niaspan at night. The aspirin significantly reduces the side effects, but if the patient still flushes, they won't feel it while sleeping.

I find it's my more highly educated patients who are most willing to go to higher dosages, because they really understand the benefits. Plus, they are more structured in their taking of medications, so are more likely to make sure to take the aspirin along with the Niaspan as recommended.

Cholesterol Combination Medication

There is a combination drug that adds Niaspan and a statin together. Called Simcor, it works the different avenues to further lower cholesterol, with Niaspan as one of the best to raise HDL and the only one to lower LPa.

There is also a combination of a statin drug and Zetia. Called Vytorin, it's been around for quite some time.

CHAPTER 40

ANTI-ANGINA DRUGS
Taking Strain off Chest Pain

There are different classes of drugs used for anti-angina. You might recall that angina is chest pain, arising from blockages creating a lack of blood flow to the heart. While this certainly can be serious, some people can get rid of their symptoms with medications.

Determining the location of the blockage is how we decide whether to use medications or go in surgically to fix it. If a blockage is in the area of the heart that will cause significant damage and heart attack if that blockage ruptures, then we do surgery. But there can be blockages in other areas of small arteries, such that even if there is a heart attack, you're not going to lose any heart muscle. In those cases, we get rid of the symptoms with medications to help blood flow, along with statins and aspirin to help prevent a heart attack.

The prototype of the angina drug is nitrates. Nitrates work by vasal dilating (opening) arteries through the smooth muscle wall of the arteries. There are several different formulations of nitrates.

There is sublingual (dissolves under the tongue) for acute attacks. If you have chest pains, it relieves the pain quickly as it immediately dilates the arteries, allowing more blood flow to the muscle and less pain.

If you're getting angina pain frequently during the day, you can take short-acting pills three times daily. There are also long-acting nitrates that are taken only once per day. They work well for the chest pains, but you can have side effects of headaches with this form, especially as you go into higher doses.

There is also a spray that can be used instead of tablets. The spray is used primarily for acute attacks of angina. Perhaps surprisingly, the spray has a longer shelf life than tablets. Normally, tablets a year old lose much of their effectiveness, and the patient is advised to inform their doctor to get new ones.

One problem with this drug is that many men with vascular disease have impotence. If they are using any drug (like Viagra) to enhance themselves sexually – they absolutely cannot use this medication for angina.

Ranexa

Nitrates have been around for over 35 years. In fact, there hasn't been a new class of angina drug in all that time since – until just a few years ago. Ranexa.

Given that I had a chance to learn and examine this product sooner than other doctors, I was able to utilize it more immediately for my patients. I do not fault other cardiologists for not embracing this as quickly, since a new drug may often end up having serious issues.

But now more and more cardiologists are utilizing it. It works differently than nitrates. Instead of functioning at the level of the vessel, it works at the *cellular level of the heart*. It relaxes the heart's muscles as it is beating, so it doesn't squeeze the artery as it pumps. This way the artery has more blood flow to the muscle of the heart.

When Ranexa initially came out, it had a *potential* side effect of bringing on arrhythmias in patients (proarrhythmia). But in thousands and thousands of patients, not one person has ever had this problem. So the FDA has recently relaxed this concern, such that Ranexa is now considered quite safe and can be used with other drugs. In fact, latest studies have shown that for people coming into a hospital with a mild heart attack, Ranexa can immediately *lower* the chance of arrhythmias – the opposite of what was initially expected.

Beneficial to Diabetics

Some studies have also shown Ranexa can work with the pancreas to lower the levels of *Hemoglobin A1c* in patients with diabetes. Hemoglobin A1c in the blood is the best marker (indicator) to see how well blood sugar is being controlled for diabetic patients. Even some drugs used specifically for diabetes aren't as effective in doing this.

Success Close to Home

At 92 years old, my wife's grandfather had numerous blockages in arteries all over this body. Even though his condition was pretty serious and I'm a cardiologist, you always want to weigh the risks of bringing a patient in for surgery.

I tend not to be overly aggressive in my approach. I think things through, rather than simply make money by doing stents on everyone. So even though he had multiple blockages and symptoms (he couldn't walk 10 yards before he had chest pains), it was risky at his age to perform surgery to open up his arteries.

So I put him on Ranexa. I've had him on this drug for three years now and he's had no pain. Today, *he walks three miles a day* without any problem. That's pretty impressive for anyone in their nineties (he's now 95), but he knows how important exercise is. This drug (and several others I have him taking) has allowed him to be active.

Other Drugs Can Help Too

There are other classes of drugs that can also help with angina, even though they're not necessarily called anti-angina drugs. They include calcium channel blockers and beta blockers.

I previously mentioned that calcium channel blockers relax the smooth cells within vessels to dilate them. Because of that function, calcium channel blockers can also be used to relieve angina symptoms.

Beta blockers work differently, by affecting "supply and demand" in the body. Just as the rule of supply and demand affects our economy – if the supply of available blood to the heart is less than what it demands, a person will have chest pain. When you have a blockage and you walk, the supply of oxygen-rich blood may remain limited, but the requirements of the heart go up. You can't supply more oxygen to the muscle, so you get pain. That's why people can have those pains when exerting themselves, but don't when sitting around.

But by lowering the muscle's need for oxygen – by lowering the heart rate and intensity of each beat – the supply you get will be adequate and you can walk longer before you reach that level when the demand is enough to cause pain. That is how beta blockers function.

CHAPTER 41

ANTI-ARRHYTHMIC DRUGS

Keeping a Steady Pace

There are several drugs that help with the abnormal electrical activity of the heart associated with arrhythmias and palpitations. They all work differently, with varying potential side effects.

Amiodarone and Multaq

The drug that cardiologists use most frequently is Amiodarone. It can affect arrhythmias occurring from the top or the lower chamber of the heart. In my practice, with people having atrial fibrillation or arrhythmias, we try to use the least amount of drugs possible. We'll try beta blockers first to see if they can maintain the heart's normal function. If that doesn't work, we can try Amiodarone, as it helps stabilize the irritation of the cells that would cause the arrhythmia.

While it works really well, Amiodarone contains iodine, which can cause people to develop thyroid problems. On extremely rare occasions – less than half of one percent – it can also cause irreversible lung damage (pulmonary fibrosis).

But recently a new drug has come out, called Multaq. This is a new formulation of Amiodarone that doesn't have iodine that can cause thyroid problems, nor can it bring on lung damage. Still, as I have already cited, no drug is perfect. Multaq is not good for people with weak hearts, such as those with diagnosed "congestive heart failure." Conversely, the original form of the drug – Amiodarone – is fine for weak hearts.

Obviously, there is no one drug that fits all. Every person is different, with different conditions and needs. That's why you want a skilled and comprehensive cardiologist to be choosing the exact right medication for you.

CHAPTER 42

BLOOD THINNERS

The Skinny on Blood Thinning

Aspirin – that common, inexpensive, over-the-counter drug that's been around since the late 1800s – continues being one of the best blood thinners out there today.

People at risk with heart disease – especially those with diabetes, or with multiple risk factors and over the age of 50, or who have already experienced a heart attack – are especially well-served by taking aspirin. For long-term usage like this, a baby (81 mg) is sufficient to get the benefit. What benefit?

Aspirin can reduce the likelihood of death. Pretty significant.

If you're having a heart attack and you take an aspirin, it is almost as good as the older thrombolytic drugs they used to give people who showed up with heart attacks. It reduces mortality by nearly *30 percent*. So as I've said earlier – if you think you are having a heart attack, in this case you want to chew a full strength (325 mg) aspirin. If you have no full strength aspirin available, chewing four baby aspirin can work too.

Aspirin is very safe. But if you have absolutely no risk factors, you don't need to take it. There's no benefit to take medications you don't need. It just another ingredient your body has to process.

Plavix and Effient

Here is a very instructive case of a drug that at first appeared to be a blessing for those with a specific condition, but turned out to have problems.

Plavix is an antiplatelet agent used to prevent blood clot formation, and as such, has been used successfully as a blood thinner along with medicated stents. But the FDA began watching Plavix for interactions with other particular drugs – all of which use the same enzyme in the liver as does Plavix, as part of their actions on the body. It was discovered if that enzyme is already being used by another drug and is not available to Plavix, the Plavix won't be effective. Someone could have a heart attack, as the vessel might close down with a blockage. This demonstrates one way that drugs can interact with each other.

Since then a new drug has come out, called Effient. It doesn't use that same liver enzyme and so doesn't have those interactions with other drugs.

Effient is actually more potent, and used for a select group of patients. Studies have shown it to lower chances of patients getting heart attacks. In fact, for patients with medicated stents, it's a 64 percent reduction compared to those people taking Plavix. Patients would only need to take this drug for one year. By that time, the lining should be forming around the stent and the person should be fine.

Coumadin

Coumadin is used as a blood thinner for several categories of people: those with deep venous thrombosis (a blood clot forming in a vein deep in the body)...or blood clots in the legs or lungs...or irregular heartbeats such as atrial fibrillation (which can cause blood clots in the left atrium chamber of the heart)...or for people with a mechanical heart valve.

Coumadin is effective, but difficult to use. It has many drug interactions. For example, Tylenol would cause Coumadin to make the blood too thin. Or a patient could get some antibiotic from their primary care doctor who doesn't question if the patient is on Coumadin, causing a severe interaction where blood thinning dramatically elevates. That can cause bleeding from his nose, gastrointestinal tract, or even within the brain.

Even some foods can affect Coumadin. Green leafy vegetables actually diminish its effect. So periodically eating a lot of salads can raise or lower the blood thinning effect. You're potentially leaving the patient at risk for a stroke.

So Coumadin is cumbersome. You have to constantly check blood work to make sure the blood is not too thin or thick.

Pradaxa

A new drug has now replaced Coumadin for patients with atrial fibrillation. You don't have to worry about interactions with other drugs, nor will food intake affect how it works.

When you take Pradaxa, you know you're getting the right amount of blood thinning and that you're protected. In the right dose, it's also more effective in preventing stroke than Coumadin.

Having said all this, it is still not a perfect drug. While the cause remains unknown, it has been noted that Pradaxa patients may be at slightly more risk for heart attack and for intestinal bleeding than those on Coumadin. But both are extremely low if the patient is monitored correctly.

It's also much easier to use. If you give this drug twice a day, you don't have to check blood levels every few days or every week anymore. It's effective within two hours of taking it. A definite improvement.

The Future of Drugs

I recently lectured that I believe medicine is still in its infancy, in both how we understand and how we treat patients.

Right now, if something is off balance or too high in one part of the body, we'll give a medication to correct it. If some area is low, we'll give something else to increase its level. But as I always say, the body is extremely complex. You can't conduct medicine like a cookbook – do this for this, that for that. The system is too interrelated. I expect that the best thing in our future will be excellent genetic engineering, such that we can create a super pill that takes every aspect of our physiologic environment in perspective.

Amazing discoveries are still ahead.

CHAPTER 43

CHOOSING A GOOD DOCTOR
Good Choices, Good Health

No matter how well-educated a patient becomes – and I'm all for patients being highly knowledgeable and proactive in their pursuit of health – no patient should go it alone. They need the assistance, guidance and expertise of a trained medical doctor.

As evidenced in this book, cardiology is a complex field, requiring immense expertise and understanding. You want to select a good cardiologist as your partner in health. A good cardiologist is up-to-date on all the most recent advancements in the field. A good cardiologist has access to the latest equipment to conduct sophisticated tests. A good cardiologist knows the most current protocols to correct issues, and understands the medications to counteract heart issues.

So the question naturally arises – how do you choose a good cardiologist? Let's examine what makes an ideal physician, as well as some misconceptions.

Pursuit of Excellence

What makes a doctor excellent is their personality, their upbringing, their educational background, their attitude toward patients and their practice, and how active they are in continued education. Surprisingly, a doctor's quality is also reflected in how much they give back to patients and community, as that shows their commitment to their profession and to others, which itself is echoed in their reputation around their workplace, and by word of mouth.

If your doctor truly loves what they do, they are a physician first, then a businessperson. Money is important since they have a responsibility to provide for their family, but that does not obscure the fact that their patients come first. They are passionate about their profession. You can pick all this up about a doctor by observation and feedback from others, as well as noticing how active they are in their field and in giving back to the community. This is the foremost criteria for a good doctor.

Taking this a step further, ask yourself if the doctor seems willing to be an "average Joe or Jill" doctor…or do they always try to keep up with the latest in their field? One way to check is to find out if the doctor is Board Certified in their field. This shows that at least they care enough to stay up-to-date, since almost all specialties require recertification at least every 10 years. Admittedly, 10 years is a very long time in cardiology, considering the constant advancements. Perhaps it's simply more telling if the doctor *isn't* Board Certified.

Another consideration is to find out if they're involved in any research, and if so, do they publish? As long as they publish, it doesn't matter if it is in a peer-reviewed journal. Even if they just write for the general media, you can rest assured that they've had to review all the latest literature and become quite informed.

You should also pay attention to their office. Is it modern? Does it have most of the latest diagnostic equipment described in this book? If not, does the doctor readily send patients somewhere so those tests can be conducted?

Misconceptions

So what are some misconceptions about determining whether someone is an excellent doctor?

Which medical school they attended really has less value than you might imagine. There are mediocre doctors from excellent big-name schools, and there are excellent doctors from mediocre medical schools.

Further, there is a false belief that if a doctor is head or chief of the department, then they must be the best. The truth is, they may or may not be the best; all that's certain is they are politically well-versed.

Certainly, academic doctors (those teaching others) are almost always exceptionally well informed about the latest literature and information, and may micro-specialize in their field more than most. They are better at treating the most difficult and rare diseases. This means if you have a very specific disease and know of an academic center that specializes in that particular malady, then by all means consult that particular center. At the same time, very knowledgeable private practice doctors are experienced in the most common disease states, as they see and deal with those conditions in very large numbers.

The Recognition Factor

Lastly, as holds true regardless of one's field of practice – success attracts success. If a doctor is successful, professional organizations will then want to affiliate with this particular doctor.

So awards from organizations are also signs that this doctor has achieved a certain distinction. But you should be careful *which* organizations are the ones giving the accolades, as some organizations are more legitimate than others. For example, Castle Connolly is one organization that recognizes doctors in various fields in the United States. It is highly respected, as it researches and rates best doctors in part by requiring multiple nominations for candidates from its base of already established "best doctors." As a member myself, I can attest to the standards they hold for all their doctors.

Though grateful to be recognized in this way, I also strongly feel you shouldn't rely on such awards 100 percent in choosing a doctor. There are many excellent doctors that have not been recognized for one reason or another.

Still, all that I've mentioned so far are good overall guidelines to helping choose a fine doctor. To further that pursuit, I want to provide a few more distinctions to consider as you make your best selection.

Bedside Manner

Let me pose a question. Which would be the more commendable: a caring, loving, competent but average doctor...or a highly intelligent, uncaring doctor?

From my phrasing, you probably sense I would suggest the former. In fact, to again quote Albert Einstein, "Most people say that it is the intellect which makes a great scientist. They are wrong: it is character."

Knowledge is a fantastic tool, but is only as good as the person employing it. Doctors need to be genuinely interested in their patients.

Along with the doctor's commitment and character, also key is how their "bedside manner" adjusts to fit various patients' needs and personalities. For example, with myself, since many patients coming to me have a degree of fear about heart health, I don't explain their condition in the same way to each one. There are many different kinds of people out there, and I've seen wildly different responses to the same information.

But after interviewing thousands and thousands of them, I have a good feel for different patients and what they can handle. Their educational background, cultural background, how they speak, how they perceive the disease process – all of these play roles in how they will respond.

With all of this in my head, I try to give what they can understand. The highly educated and computer savvy generally get many more details. For others who might have less education, but culturally have more respect for doctors, I try to be more of a father figure as I explain to them what is going on. But I may not go into quite as much detail as I explain what I think is best for them to do.

If they are neither well-educated nor have cultural respect for doctors – it can be very difficult to convince them of their situation. Sometimes they just don't want to do *anything*.

Frankly, there are also those who simply don't care. They smoke. They overeat. They've already wrecked their body. If they refuse to take a surgical step I might recommend, then I suggest we at least start some medication to help protect them.

Recognizing a Patient's Support System

What also separates the average from really good doctors is their having a greater feel for the disease process.

The better doctors usually have a pretty strong sense of how sick someone is. Do they have something that we should act on within a few days? Is a month fine to wait? Or do they need to be admitted to the hospital immediately?

You might be surprised, but included in this decision is knowing their support system. If they are well-educated and surrounded by nurturing family and friends, we are more comfortable if they go home and let us know if any further symptoms arise. Obviously that is also dependent on their disease and its likely progression, plus their use of some medication we might be prescribing. But if we feel there isn't a support system for them, then we may be inclined to get them in sooner for more invasive testing and possible surgery.

A Thinking Doctor

Though this may seem obvious, you also want a doctor who *thinks*. You don't want somebody just following preset protocols that they apply to everyone.

To illustrate, let me tell you something that might be surprising: the body has ways of overcoming what we're doing.

What do I mean by that?

Sometimes a medication that's initially effective becomes less so over time as the body re-compensates. An example might be we might block one receptor, but the body finds another mechanism to work around it. Unfortunately, when a medication that was effective no longer works, some doctors take the position, "Well, if it's stopped working at this dosage…I'll just give a higher dose."

Not always the best approach.

It is better to put everything in perspective. What has changed? What other medications might do a better job from this point forward? These attitudes reflect differences between an acceptable doctor and a much better one. I'm not simply speaking of myself here. There are many excellent doctors in every field of medicine. But not all doctors are the same, even if they share similar degrees from similar universities.

The truth is, some doctors are excellent in just rote memory and knowledge. They practice medicine like a cookbook: you have this symptom, so we give you this for it. If you have a different symptom, then we give what is called for to solve that. They're not analytical about it. They don't put information together to discover new ways specific to a patient's needs that might not be a "textbook case."

But no two people are the same. Every patient has their own disease process. One person's responses can be quite different from those of other patients with the same disease. You have to take so much into perspective when you treat a patient.

Fortunately, the doctors using this "textbook" approach are not great in number. In general, most doctors treat analytically. I suppose it's no different than any other field. You have the better ones and the not as good. But in medicine, you're dealing with someone's health and their life. While I'm not expecting this book will change the way some doctors practice, I do hope it will change how *patients* look at their health, at medicine, and at what they expect and want from a physician.

Let me give an example. I just treated a 48-year-old man with full-blown hypertension and high cholesterol. But he doesn't have any symptoms, nor does he want to take any drugs because he doesn't believe in medication. He simply wants to exercise and improve his diet. So after a period of time, he comes back for another checkup. He still has high blood pressure. He still has high cholesterol.

Rather than push him harder toward medication, I had him tested on the cardiovascular profiler (CVP) in my office. It revealed an abnormality that told me his arteries were not functioning in a healthy manner. That's very important to know. The first thing that goes bad in cardiovascular disease is that your arteries aren't healthy. Then you're more prone to develop blockages.

Knowing his personality and his intentions, I clearly explained to him, "You are at the start of this health 'cascade.' A stress-echo shows that you do not have tight blockages, but you do have the beginning signs of problems because of your high cholesterol. If you had high cholesterol, but the CVP showed that you were normal, then I would say maybe you can hold off medication and just diet and exercise. But we now know that you have artery issues along with high cholesterol. You need to take cholesterol medication. Then I'll bring you back and retest you – and prove to you that once your cholesterol goes down, your arteries improve."

He agreed to take medication, and when he returned and we retested – the arteries were functioning better. He was convinced. I've done this with numerous other patients, always with positive effects. This same approach of testing – taking medications and retesting – can be used with CIMT and CRP tests as well, for patients that may initially be resistant to starting medications.

Good Doctor, Good Patient

Clearly, you must be wise in selecting your doctors. But once you have done your homework and found your doctor of choice – then you also need to accept and trust their advice. You want a good doctor, *and* you want to be a good patient. You need to listen and follow their guidance. After all, it is *your* health and well-being that you both are trying to improve.

CHAPTER 44

AMERICAN COLLEGE OF CARDIOLOGY

A Medical Society

My last chapter cited that excellent doctors stay atop the latest developments in their field. I also declared that successful doctors most likely are part of successful professional organizations. In actuality, these two truths are interrelated.

As stated early in this book, cardiology is perhaps the most rapidly changing field in medicine. With so many conducting research and new discoveries occurring around the world, you might wonder how all this new information is reviewed and disseminated to doctors.

The American College of Cardiology is the leader in bringing together guidelines for the aspects and disease entities in cardiology. It creates all the educational materials and latest findings that are distributed to cardiologists. At its annual conference, over *37,000* people attend from across the globe – pretty much everyone. That's not to say those from Europe and elsewhere around the globe don't have their own meetings, but their members come to us as well. We host the seminars that present the most current information and research.

I strongly feel that doctors should get actively involved (beyond just paying dues) within the Society. They will not only benefit from the most up-to-date research, but can also make a difference in the profession. I endorse this with assurance, as I have served as a council representative, and as Chair of Media Relations at the American College of Cardiology for California.

I've met many terrific doctors through my work with this society. As described in the last chapter, hallmarks of those doctors are a passion for their work, learning the newest developments – plus giving back to the community. Involvement with this organization is one avenue for doctors to do this. As example, our organization has a theme every year. Recently, Dr. Alfred Bove, past president of American College of Cardiology, declared our theme "The Year of the Patient." The focus was educating patients about heart disease and the different ways cardiologists can help them. My presentation was one of the first dedicated to this theme and kicked off that year's event. I explained the Sudden Death in Athletes program that I developed in California, where I put together an alliance of hospitals to donate defibrillators to high schools. Plus, once having gotten that in place, I began accelerating the program to find ways for funding donations of defibrillators to *all* the high schools in California.

I am very grateful to the California Chapter of the American College of Cardiology, and past president Gordon Fung, MD, for their absolute support of this project. Hopefully my presentation will encourage other doctors to do similarly where they live and practice. I don't bring this up to pat myself on the back. I simply want you to recognize the kinds of actions you might see from dedicated, passionate doctors.

One can make a difference in many ways. Being part of an organization such as this, you can get involved in the politics of cardiology too. Now you may wonder, "Politics...in cardiology?" Yes, and by understanding those politics, a doctor can make big differences not only for the society, but also for humanity at large.

For instance, laws and regulations are formulated in Congress that affect the treatments for Medicare patients. Yet most congressional representatives really don't understand the issues in relationship to cardiology care. They're legislators, not physicians. Cardiologists know what's truly best for patients, and we're able to explain the ways that we should be practicing medicine to maintain quality of care for the patient. At the same time, we're protecting the rights of patients so their costs don't go up.

The American College of Cardiology has gained significant respect from lawmakers, its own members, and patients, as a highly caring and professional organization. In fact, the current president of ACC, Dr. Ralph Brindis, has named this The Year of Professionalism, encouraging ACC members to maintain the highest possible professionalism in their practice of cardiovascular medicine.

CHAPTER 45

BELIEF IN SCIENCE

Merging of Worlds

As much as we've advanced our science, there are still mysteries in medicine, as in life. Some of them continue to puzzle the most sophisticated doctors and scientists in the world.

One of those is why certain patients survive and others do not. They each could face the same serious medical issues, receive the identical treatments…and some will thrive while some won't.

It is perhaps natural to speculate there may be realms beyond medicine yet to be understood. One clue may lie in studies conducted where prayers were performed for certain patients in a hospital and not for others. From that act alone – it was found that those who had prayers done on their behalf did significantly *better* than those who didn't.

This adds support to there being a spiritual aspect to health and recovery we've not fully grasped.

In a way, this quandary parallels a baby's development in the womb. The baby is establishing its organs so it can survive in this life, though the brain is not mature enough to understand the concept of what this life is. All they know is their experience in this nice, warm environment of the womb, yet they hear sounds from the "outside world." They know something is going on out there, but there's no way they can know what. Yet all the time, they are developing faculties so they can survive in this life.

In a similar manner, while we are in this world, we may be trying to develop our next page of life, by having necessary experiences and growing our spiritual realm. Perhaps to be ready for *our* next world, that is presently beyond our capacity to understand.

As I said, a mystery of life. Even Einstein stated, "The more I learn, the more I realize I don't know." Most scientists do not believe in God, since they cannot use the scientific method to prove its existence. Yet, the greatest scientist of our time, Einstein, has been quoted as saying that he believes in a higher being, but he just cannot define it.

Of Two Worlds

My being raised in the Bahá'í faith has certainly helped shaped me as a person. One of the good things about the Bahá'í faith is that it teaches harmony between science and religion. Sometimes those too much into religion become superstitious. Others too deep into science become fixated only on the physical.

I clearly allow credence to a spiritual world that we may not yet comprehend, but I am also a scientist. Once you get into science, you always have to *prove, prove, prove.* I feel you must have a balance.

So while acknowledging there are things beyond our knowing, I believe 100 percent that you have to see a competent physician when you are sick. *Use what has been learned through science and technology* to help get you better. This knowledge has come through to doctors for a purpose. Don't close your eyes to it and say, "I'm just going to pray till I get well."

I add to this again that you also *pay attention*. Even to things you might not understand. Perhaps some of us might sense something is amiss, without knowing why we feel that. On a more tangible level, I'll remind that the body is exquisitely designed to offer you clues when something is wrong. When you're short of breath...pay attention. When you feel palpitations in your chest...take notice. A pain anywhere in the body can be a clue to something needing to be addressed.

Some clues can only be uncovered or understood by going to your doctor and conducting specific tests. How fortunate are we, that there are traits and symptoms – and tests that can measure them – when something unseen is occurring so we can mend it.

All aspects are important. Good medical treatment, as well as prayer from the spiritual realm. I've seen too many cases in my own practice that remain a puzzle as to why some people do better than others. The belief in the spiritual seems to have an influence too. This larger view really illuminates how I treat patients.

CHAPTER 46

THE FUTURE

Roads Ahead

Good health is a partnership. It's an alliance between you and your physician. Between your physician and those on the forefronts of research. And between your mind and your own body.

Only you are with yourself all of the time. Only you will first witness, feel or even sense when some change might be occurring. Only you can alert your doctor.

It also is only you who can create a lifestyle supportive of fantastic health. Of a great future. Eating healthfully. Exercising. Visiting your doctor and taking medications when needed. Only you can think good thoughts. All contribute to positive health.

Physicians and cardiologists are committed to helping you. That is why we came into our professions. Trust me, cardiology isn't an easy science. Staying on top of latest developments, on top of your patient's needs, takes serious commitment. One doesn't enter this field professionally looking for an easy ride. We want to help. And we can. As said before, the science of cardiology is more advanced now than at anytime in history. We can do things today only dreamed of ten or twenty years ago.

Yet as sophisticated as we are, I feel we are still in our infancy. I am filled with awe as I envision where we may be headed. At the moment, it appears genetic engineering, manipulation and treatment will dramatically alter the future of medicine. Stem cell research is looking to be tremendously auspicious for patients. Helping regenerate organs as naturally as possible, rather than using prosthetics or mechanics to mend them.

All of this will change the way we practice medicine. Personally, I am very much looking forward to it. We shall all be beneficiaries.

Wishing you the best in life and in health, I hope this book has given you a deeper understanding and appreciation of the remarkable body you've been given. Treat it with respect. Cherish its gifts.

Be grateful for life.

Index

A

A-1 Milano gene, 122
ABI (ankle-brachial test), 130–131
acceptance, stages of, 149–150
ACE (angiotensin-converting
    enzyme) inhibitors, 68, 158,
    188–189
adrenergic drive, 193
adult-onset diabetes. *see* diabetes
A-fib (atrial fibrillation), 45–48
alcohol use
    benefits of, 85
    dangers of, 46
Aliskiren, 190, 191
American College of Cardiology,
    22–23, 167, 225–227, 235
Amiodarone, 211–212
Amsterdam, Erza, 20, 21
angina
    causes, 41–42
    typical symptoms, 114–115
    women's symptoms, 156
angina drugs
    beta blockers, 210
    calcium channel blockers, 210
    nitrates, 207–208
    Ranexa, 208–209
angiograms
    computed tomography (CT), 139
    shortfalls of, 162, 172
    for stent placement, 140
angiotensin receptor blockers
    (ARB), 189
angiotensin-converting enzyme
    (ACE) inhibitors, 68, 158,
    188–189
ankle-brachial test (ABI), 130–131

antibiotics
    and dental work, 61–62
    drug interactions, 215
    and Strep throat, 63–64
antiplatelet drugs, 214
aortic dissection, 42
aortic stenosis, 42
ARB (angiotensin receptor
    blockers), 189
arrhythmias
    caffeine and, 13
    diagnosis of, 127, 133, 145–146
    drugs for, 211–212
    explained, 43–45
    A-fib, 45–48
    mitral valve prolapse, 61
    pacemakers and, 52–54
    sudden cardiac death, 167–169
arterial spasms, 159–160
arteries
    aortic dissection, 42
    blockages, 41–42
    bypass surgery, 143–144
    "hardening of the arteries," 37
    spasms, 159–160
    "torn arteries," 42
arthritis
    CRP level in, 124–125
    Lovaza and, 72, 203–204
    risk of CVD, 71
aspirin
    81 mg "baby" aspirin, 213
    during a heart attack, 117, 176
    with Niaspan, 205
    and stents, 143
atherosclerosis
    diagnosis of, 129, 131
    effect of smoking on, 111

235

explained, 37
historical perspective of, 7–8
inflammation in, 60
and nitric oxide, 94–95
and PAD, 115, 130
risk factors, 87, 89
and sleep apnea, 109–110
athletes' heart health, 167–173
atrial fibrillation (A-fib), 45–48
atrium, 44
Automatic Internal Cardiac
   Defibrillator (AICD), 145–147
AV node, 44, 46
Azor, 190–191

B

Bahá'í faith, 19, 230–231
balloon angioplasty, 141
bare metal stents, 143
bedside manner, 220–221
Benazepril, 190–191
Benicar, 190–191
beta blockers
   for angina, 210
   for A-fib, 46
   how they work, 192–194
   for mitral valve prolapse, 61
bile acid sequestrants, 200–201
BioZ Impedance Cardiography
   (ICG), 134
blockages
   arterial, 32–33, 41–42
   kidney, 37–38
   symptoms of, 114–115
blood clots. *see also* hypertension
   drugs for, 213–216
   formation of, 46–47
   plaque erosion and, 159
blood pressure
   explained, 27–29
   RAAS (hormone system),
      29–30, 187–188

salt use and, 86–87
stress hormones and, 103
blood tests, 33, 123–125
blood thinners, 47, 213–216
Board Certification, 218
bradycardia, 51–52
"broken heart," 162–163
"butterflies in my heart," 49
bypass surgery, 143–144
Bystolic, 193–194

C

caffeine, 13–14, 103
calcium channel blockers
   for angina, 210
   for A-fib, 46
   how they work, 191–192
calcium score, 160–161
cardiac defibrillator. *see*
   defibrillators
cardiologists
   academia vs. private practice, 22
   choosing a doctor, 217–224
   comprehensiveness of, 3–5, 9
   diagnostic approach, 137–138, 140
   electrophysiologists, 43
   interventionalists, 43
   preparing for office visits, 119–125
   treatment approach, 149–151
cardiology
   American College of Cardiology,
      22–23, 167, 225–227, 235
   recent developments in, 11–15
cardiomyopathy, 145–146
cardiopulmonary resuscitation
   (CPR), 168, 170
cardiovascular disease (CVD)
   cardiology and, 9
   definition of, 11–12
   diagnostic approach, 137–140
   prevalence of, 7–8
   risk factors, 122–123

symptoms of, 113–118
Cardiovascular Profiler (CVP), 131–132
Cardizem, 191–192
Carotid Intima Media Thickness (CIMT), 128–130, 161
Castle Connolly, 219–220
cell phones, pacemakers and, 54
chest pains. *see* angina
cholesterol
  components of, 32–34
  dietary control, 81–85
  educating your doctor, 34–35
  healthy vs. unhealthy, 31–32
  levels in women, 160
  optimum, 33, 34, 198–199
cholesterol drugs
  absorption inhibitors, 201–202
  bile acid sequestrants, 201
  combination therapies, 205
  fenofibrates, 202–203
  niacin, 204–205
  omega-3 fatty acids, 72, 203–204
  statins, 197–200
  treatment approach, 198–199
Cialis, 179–181
CIMT (Carotid Intima Media Thickness), 128–130, 161
Coenzyme Q10 (CoQ10), 200
collateral circulation, 39
congestive heart failure, 55, 115
continuous positive airway pressure device (CPAP), 110
CoQ10 (Coenzyme Q10), 200
Coreg, 194
coronary artery bypass surgery, 143–144
coronary CTA, 139
coronary disease. *see* cardiovascular disease (CVD)
coronary reactivity, 159–160
cortisol, 103, 105–106

Coumadin, 47, 214–215
Cozaar, 189
CPAP (continuous positive airway pressure device), 110
CPR (cardiopulmonary resuscitation), 168
C-reactive protein (CRP), 124–125
Crestor, 68–69, 199
CT angiogram (CTA), 139
CVD (cardiovascular disease). *see* cardiovascular disease (CVD)
CVP (Cardiovascular Profiler), 131–132

D

defibrillators
  Automatic Internal Cardiac Defibrillator (AICD), 145–147
  how they work, 169
  portable automatic defibrillators, 170–171
dental work, and heart health, 61–62
DES (drug-eluting stents), 142
diabetes
  cholesterol guidelines in, 65–66
  connection to heart disease, 65
  medications for, 68–69
  metabolic syndrome and, 66–67
  and PAD, 39
  type 1 vs. type 2, 66–67
diagnostic tests
  angiograms, 139, 162, 172
  ankle-brachial test (ABI), 130–131
  BioZ Impedance Cardiography (ICG), 134
  blood tests, 123–125
  Cardiovascular Profiler (CVP), 131–132
  Carotid Intima Media Thickness (CIMT), 128–130

echocardiogram, 127–128
ejection fraction, 145–146
EKG, 127
Electron Beam Computerized Tomography (EBCT), 134–135
Microvolt T-Wave Alternans (MTWA), 133–134
transesophageal echo (TEE), 47
treadmill test, 138–139
VAP lipoprotein analysis, 33, 123
diastolic pressure, 27
diet. *see* nutrition
dihydropyridines, 192
Diovan, 190–191
direct renin inhibitors (DRI), 190
diuretics, 190, 194–195
drug-eluting stents (DES), 142

E

EBCT (Electron Beam Computerized Tomography), 134–135
echocardiograms, 127–128
Effient, 214
ejection fraction, 145–146
electrocardiogram (EKG), 127, 168
Electron Beam Computerized Tomography (EBCT), 134–135
electrophysiologists (EP), 43
endocarditis, and gum disease, 60–62
endorphins, 108–109
energy drinks, dangers of, 13–14
EP (electrophysiologists), 43
erectile dysfunction (ED)
beta blockers and, 193–194
and heart disease, 178–181
and nitrates, 208
estrogen, and heart disease, 12

exercise
appropriate goals for, 95–96
benefits of athletics, 171–172
effect on heart health, 93–94
effect on hormone levels, 94–95
effect on stress, 103
maximum heart rate, 96
as predictor of survival, 90
Exforge, 190–191

F

family history
and cholesterol, 32
and heart disease, 120–122
fenofibrates, 69, 202–203
fetal nutrition, effect on heart health, 165–166
fibrinogen, 124
"fight or flight syndrome," 193
fish oil. *see* omega-3 fatty acids
flavonoids, 85
fluttering feeling, 49
Framingham Risk Assessment, 161–162

G

gastric bypass surgery, 90–91
Gemfibrozil, 202–203
genetic engineering, 216
genetics, 32, 120–122
ginseng, 14
goal setting, 97–99
green tea, 86
guarana, 14
gum disease
endocarditis and, 60–62
inflammation in, 59–60
as predictor of heart disease, 59

H

"hardening of the arteries," 37
HDL cholesterol, 32–34

heart
  beats per day, 15
  embryologic development of, 1
  A-fib, 45
  structure and operation of,
    43–45
heart attack, symptoms of,
  116–117
heart disease. *see* cardiovascular
  disease
heart health
  cardiologist's role in, 3–5
  choosing a doctor, 217–224
  future possibilities for, 233–234
  importance to happiness, 1–2
  knowledge as power, 172–173
  lifestyle choices and, 79–80
  recent developments in, 11–15
  recognizing symptoms, 113,
    118, 231
  setting goals for, 97–99
heart valves, 42, 61–62
hemoglobin A1c, 209
homocysteine levels, 123–124
hormone levels
  effect of exercise on, 94–95
  estrogen, 12
  and microvessel disease, 158
  RAAS system, 29–30, 187–188
  replacement therapy, 155–156
  during stress, 103–104
hydration, 14
hypertension. *see also* blood
    pressure
  and aortic dissection, 42
  defined, 27
  and A-fib, 46
  genetic origin of, 165
  and kidney function, 37–38
  and obesity, 121
  and salt, 86–88

vitamin D deficiency and,
    163–164
  "white coat hypertension," 120
hypertension drugs
  ACE inhibitors, 188–189
  ARB, 189
  beta blockers, 192–194
  calcium channel blockers,
    191–192
  combination drugs, 190–191
  dihydropyridines, 192
  diuretics, 194–195
  DRI, 190
  RAAS (hormone system) and,
    187–188
hyperthyroidism, and A-fib, 46

I

impotence. *see* erectile
    dysfunction (ED)
indigestion pain, misdiagnosis of,
  41
internal cardiac defibrillator,
  145–147
interventionalist cardiologists, 43
iodine, 211–212
IPG (Bioz Impedance
    Cardiography), 134

J

juvenile diabetes. *see* diabetes

K

kidney function, 37–38

L

lactic acid, in angina, 42
L-Arginine, 179
LDL cholesterol
  in atherosclerosis, 94–95
  relation to HDL, 32–33
"left bundle," 44–45

Left Ventricular Assist Device
(LVAD), 99
Levitra, 179–181
Lipitor, 68–69, 199
liver damage, 200
Lotrel, 190–191
Lovastatin, 68–69
Lovaza, 72, 84, 203–204
LP(a) cholesterol, 33
LVAD (Left Ventricular Assist
Device), 99

M

Mandibular Advancement
Device, 110
Manshadi, Ramin
American College of
Cardiology, 225–227
benefits of athletics, 171–172
birth and early life of, 17–20
challenges overcome, 97–99
choice of cardiology, 20–21
philosophy of life, 23, 229–231
professional affiliations, 22–23,
235
service in Honduras, 73–77
thirst for knowledge, 23–24
maximum heart rate, 96
medical schools, 219
medicated stents, 142
medications. *see also individual
names*
anti-angina, 201–210
anti-arrhythmic, 211–212
anti-hypertensive, 187–195
benefits of drug research,
183–184
blood thinners, 213–216
cholesterol lowering, 197–205
choosing the best, 186, 199,
222–223

combination therapies,
185–186, 190–191
Mediterranean Diet, 82–85
metabolic syndrome
diabetes and, 66–67
and sleep apnea, 110
Micardis, 190–191
microvessel disease, 157–158
Microvolt T-Wave Alternans
(MTWA), 133–134
microwaves, pacemakers and,
53–54
mini-strokes, symptoms of, 47
mitral valve prolapse, and dental
work, 61–62
mitral valve stenosis, and Strep
throat, 64
morbid obesity, 90–91
MTWA (Microvolt T-Wave
Alternans), 133–134
Multaq, 211–212

N

niacin
and LPa, 33
vs. Niaspan, 204–205
vs. Zetia, 201–202
Niaspan, 204–205
nitrates
for angina, 207–208
Viagra interaction, 180
nitric oxide, 94–95
nodes, heart, 44
norepinephrine, 103
Norvasc, 190–191
nuclear imaging evaluation, 139
nutrition
effect on heart health, 8
green tea, 86
healthy eating goals, 81–82
omega-3 fatty acids, 72, 83–84,
203–204

pediatric concerns, 87–88
red wine, 85
salt, 86–87

O

obesity
 connection to heart disease,
  89–90
 and metabolic syndrome, 66–67
 morbid obesity, 90–91
 prevalence of, 89
 women's heart issues, 163
obstructive sleep apnea, 109–110
omega-3 fatty acids, 72, 83–84,
  203–204
optimism, 164–165
oral hygiene. *see* gum disease

P

PAC (Premature Atrial Complex),
 49
pacemakers, 52–54
PAD (peripheral arterial disease).
 see peripheral arterial disease
 (PAD)
palpitations
 bradycardia, 51–52
 congenital, 50–51
 pacemakers and, 52–54
 Premature Atrial Complex
  (PAC), 49
 Premature Ventricular
  Complex (PVC), 50
 stress hormones and, 103
 symptoms of, 49
peripheral arterial disease (PAD)
 causes, 39
 effect of smoking on, 111
 explained, 37–38
 and kidney function, 38
 symptoms of, 115
 tests for, 130–131

vs. varicose veins, 40
phosphodiesterase inhibitors,
  179–181
physical activity. *see* exercise
plaque, 37, 60
plaque erosion, 159, 197–198
Plavix, 214
portable automatic defibrillators,
  167–171
Pradaxa, 215
Pravachol, 68–69, 199
prayer, power of, 229–231
pregnancy, medications to avoid,
  189
Premature Atrial Complex (PAC),
 49
Premature Ventricular Complex
 (PVC), 50
proarrhythmias, 209
Propanol, 192–193
pulmonary fibrosis, 211
pulse
 in bradycardia, 51–52
 heartbeats per day, 15
 normal vs. abnormal, 45
 in SVT, 50
PVC (Premature Ventricular
 Complex), 50

R

RAAS (renin-angiotensin-
 aldosterone system), 29–30,
 187–188
RAAS blockade drugs
 ACE inhibitors, 188–189
 ARB drugs, 189
renin inhibitors, 190
Ranexa, 208–209
rebound reflex, 141
red wine, 85
remodeling, 160–161

renin-angiotensin-aldosterone
system (RAAS), 29–30,
187–188
Reynolds Risk Score, 162
"right bundle," 44–45

S

salt, 86–87
security screenings, pacemakers
and, 53
sex
and coronary conditions, 177
erectile dysfunction (ED),
178–179
L-Arginine, 179
phosphodiesterase inhibitors
and, 179–181
side effects, of medications,
184–185, 199–200
"silent killer," 113
Simcor, 205
Simvastatin, 199
sinus node, 44
sleep
importance to heart health,
107–108
improving the quality of,
108–109
sleep apnea, 109–110
smoking
effect on atherosclerosis, 111
effect on longevity, 112
and PAD, 39
spirituality, power of, 229–231
sports drinks, dangers of, 13–14
statin drugs
benefits of, 197–198
in diabetes, 68–69
side effects of, 199–200
stents, 38, 141–143

Strep throat, and heart disease,
62–64
stress
acupuncture and, 104
beta blockers and, 193
causes of, 101–102
coronary reactivity and,
159–160
cortisol, 105–106
effect on heart health, 29–30
hormone levels and, 103
interpersonal relationships
and, 104–105
psychosomatic pain from,
102–103
releases for, 102
sleep loss and, 108–109
stress test, 138–139
sudden cardiac death
portable automatic
defibrillators, 170–171
prevention, 168–169
screening for, 14–15
stages of, 167–168
surviving, 169
weighing risks of, 171–172
support systems, 221–222
supraventricular tachycardia
(SVT), 45, 50
symptoms
atypical in women, 41, 114–115,
156
of congestive heart failure, 115
of coronary disease, 114–115
of heart attack, 116–117
of peripheral arterial disease
(PAD), 115
recognizing, 113, 118, 231
summary of, 116
of valve disease, 115
systolic pressure, 27

T

tachycardia, 45
taurine, 14
TEE (transesophageal echo), 47
Tekturna, 190
thrombolytic drugs, 213–216
thyroid disease, 46
tobacco use. *see* smoking
"torn arteries," 42
total cholesterol, 32–33
transesophageal echo (TEE), 47
treadmill test, 138–139
triglycerides, 32–33
Trilipix, 202–203
Twynsta, 190–191

V

Valsartan, 191
Valturna, 191
valves
    disease symptoms, 115
    heart, 42, 61
    in veins, 40
VAP lipoprotein analysis test, 33,
    123
varicose veins, 39–40
Verapamil, 191–192
Viagra, 179–181
vitamin D, 163–164
Vitamin E, 185
Vytorin, 199, 205

W

Welchol, 200, 201

wine, red, 85
winter coronary risks, 175–176
women's heart issues
    atypical symptoms, 41,
        114–115, 156
    "broken heart," 162–163
    calcium score, 160–161
    cholesterol levels, 160
    CIMT results, 161
    coronary reactivity, 159–160
    deaths from CVD, 11–12
    disease predisposition, 153–154
    effect of smoking on, 112
    estrogen and, 12
    fetal nutrition, 165–166
    Framingham Risk Assessment,
        161–162
    hormone replacement therapy,
        155–156
    medication during pregnancy,
        189
    microvascular dysfunction,
        157–158
    obesity, 163
    optimism and, 164–165
    plaque erosion, 159
    Reynolds Risk Score, 162
    SVT, 50
    vitamin D deficiency, 163–164

Z

Zetia, 201–202
Zocor, 199

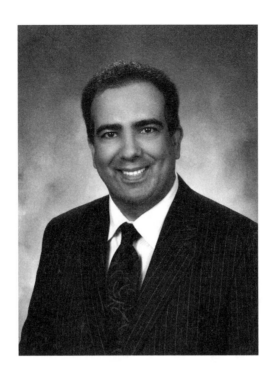

Dr. Ramin Manshadi is a multi-boarded Interventional Cardiologist treating patients from prevention to intervention. He entered the field of medicine primarily to provide humanitarian services. Because of his selfless dedication, he has been honored with awards from many reputable organizations, including America's Top Doctors from Castle Connolly, Consumers Research and *U.S. News & World Report,* Young Physician of the Year from San Joaquin Medical Society, Future Leader Award from American College of Cardiology, California Chapter among others. He complements his private practice with Academic Medicine and currently serves as Associate Clinical Professor at UC Davis Medical Center, Clinical Professor at University of the Pacific, and serves as the Chair of Media Relations for American College of Cardiology, California Chapter.

www.drmanshadi.com
R.Manshadi@drmanshadi.com